"A GATEWAY TO THE 21ST CENTURY OF MEDICINE"

THE
RESTORATION
OF THE
HUMAN BODY

[IN 7 PARTS]

SECOND EDITION

RESTORE YOUR BODY - OPTIMIZE YOUR HEALTH

D1384466

SERGEY A. DZUGAN, MD, PhD
KONSTANTINE S. DZUGAN

The Restoration of the Human Body

in Seven Parts

The Restoration of the Human Body in Seven Parts

This book is dedicated to my family: my wife, Yelena, and my three sons, Sergey, Alexander, and Konstantine.

Table of Contents

Foreword

Peter G. Fedor-Freybergh, MD, PhD, Dr. h.c. mult.
Obstetrician, Gynecologist, Child Psychiatrist,
Psychiatrist, Psychotherapist

Jenny Beatriz Loria Muñoz, MD
Director of Aesthetic Services

Professor George Birkmayer MD, PhD
Professor of Medicine and Medical Director

Peter G. Fedor-Freybergh, MD, PhD, Dr. h.c multi. Obstetrician, Gynecologist, Psychiatrist, Child Psychiatrist, Psychotherapist

"We stay on the intellectual shoulders of the giants of medicine from past days, and we are able to see further than they did only because they helped us to do so."
Claude Bernard

"Imagination is more important than knowledge."
Albert Einstein

The new book by Dr. Sergey Dzugan that you hold in your hands, *The Restoration of the Human Body*, is an excellent, most unique masterpiece, a gateway to the 21st century of medicine. The book is written in an easy-going way like a pirouette by a prima ballerina, seemingly so light and easy, but yet conveying the highest professionalism, training and thorough knowledge of each detail involved. It is an elegant piece of work of a highly scientific level, and at the same time it is understandable, full of common sense, even amusing, written both for professionals and laymen alike—a book for the intelligent reader. This book is a must and should be possessed by libraries, university libraries, and bookshelves of private persons, even as a bedside pleasure.

I am proud and happy that I was bestowed with the honor of writing a foreword to this book. I remember meeting Dr. Dzugan for the first time at the International Anti-Aging

Conference in Milan. After his brilliant lecture, the overwhelmed audience rushed out to get his signature on his previous book, *Your Blood Doesn't Lie!*, which was a fascinating reading for me, as well.

Sergey Dzugan's book discusses at length the science behind physiologic decline, how it can be restored, and about the art of aging, presenting enough information in the best way possible so that the reader can have a better understanding of how our bodies work. A question is posed: "How does the restoration of human physiology work?" Dzugan's answer is, "By natural approach," which takes into account a multitude of subsystems that need to be fixed so that the body is rejuvenated to the point of what it was we enjoyed in our twenties.

One of the quotes to this foreword is by Claude Bernard, who, besides being one of the greatest physiologists of all time, has also seen the close connections between science and art. Claude Bernard believed that the artist can find more stable ground in science and that the scientist may generate a safe intuition from art. He was convinced that if physiology progressed long enough, there would be an understanding between the poet, the philosopher, and the physiologist.

The human life should be considered as an indivisible continuum in which each of the developmental stages is equally important, all the stages interdependent and inseparable from the individual's whole life continuum. In this continuum, the individual represents the indivisible entity of all functions on the physiological (or physical), psychological, and social levels. The physical, biochemical, endocrinological, immunological, and psychological processes represent a whole that cannot be divided.

The transdisciplinary and integrative aspect of sciences and their entrance into the 21st century is the true vision of our common efforts. In this light, is also how I see this new book by Sergey Dzugan. Reading it gave me much pleasure and inspiration, and I warmly recommend it to the broad public of both professionals and interested laymen.

I wish this book a successful journey!

****

Peter G. Fedor-Freybergh is Obstetrician, Gynecologist, Psychiatrist, Child Psychiatrist, Psychotherapist.
Professor in Psychoneuroendocrinology, Child and Adolescent Psychiatry.
Professor in Prenatal and Perinatal Psychology and Medicine.
Editor-in-Chief of NEUROENDOCRINOLOGY LETTERS.
Co-Editor in Chief of BIOGENIC AMINES.
Founder and Editor-in-Chief of INT J OF PRENATAL & PERINATAL PSYCHOLOGY & MEDICINE.
Co-Chief Editor of ACTIVITAS NERVOSA SUPERIOR REDIVIVA.
Honorary Life President: International Society of Prenatal and Perinatal Psychology and Medicine.

Jenny Beatriz Loria Muñoz, MD.
Medical Director
Med Spa de Cancun, Mexico

It was a pleasure to have met Dr. Dzugan and much more of an honor to be one of the people to provide a foreword. As a medical doctor, I have been exposed to general, aesthetic, and "anti-aging" medicine, but the knowledge that I have received by experimenting with this horizon through the eyes of Dr. Dzugan, for me, has been "the missing link" - that has joined all my previous studies, investigations, and days of hard work. I think this book is an opportunity for anyone who really wants to learn and understand the human body and its physiology.

To me, the human body is like a puzzle, which now makes more sense thanks to Dr. Dzugan's guidelines (which he so kindly chooses to share). I feel more secure and confident that now I'm "really preventing and healing," which was always my goal when I was a very young woman and had chosen this profession. My recommendation to everyone, especially my colleagues, is to read this book and unlock the door to your new horizon.

It is logical! It is Physiology! It is The Restoration of the Human Body!

****

Jenny Beatriz Loria Muñoz is the Medical Director of Wellness and Cosmetic Laser Center, Med Spa de Cancun, Mexico.

Professor George Birkmayer, MD, PhD

This book is exciting in many senses. It provides a lot of very valuable information for health-conscious people. Dr. Dzugan describes difficult physiological processes in simple terms by using comparisons to actions in our daily lives. For me, most importantly, he sweeps away certain dogmas of mainstream medicine, e.g., that lowering cholesterol will improve your health. All his arguments are based on solid scientific evidence.

In Part I, "On the History of Medicine and the Nature of Disease," Dr. Dzugan points out that "medicine has roots deep in prehistory." It was interesting to learn that even animals eat certain plants for their health problems. What Egyptian, Persian and Greek healers were able to accomplish with their methods for their patients and what impact this had on modern medicine is described in a most entertaining way.

In Part II, "On the Pitfalls of Conventional Medicine," Dr. Dzugan explains with logical arguments why health care is not free and what should be done to make it free again. His statement, "The problem with the current conventional medical model is that it does not focus on the actual root cause of many diseases and health conditions, but instead goes after the symptoms," is 100 percent true. Hence, new approaches should be considered. Dr. Dzugan does outline this new philosophy in his book.

In Part III, "On the Nature and Effects of Hormones," we learn of the importance of hormones and their precursors, such as DHEA, pregnenolone, and testosterone. Dr. Dzugan clarifies why bioidentical hormones are the best physiological option regarding hormone deficiencies and why synthetic hormones like particular estrogens can increase the risk for cancer development. High testosterone levels are associated with decreased prostate cancer risk, and high levels prior to the occurrence of prostate cancer resulted in improved survival rates. This is really good news for many people.

In Part IV, "On the Nature of the Restorative Approach," the reader learns about Dr. Dzugan's concept of his diagnostic and therapeutic approach. I fully agree with his philosophy "that any human being is an individual and should be treated individually." He does not put all people in one pot and does not treat them all with the same blood pressure medications and statins.

In Part V, "On the Nature of Cholesterol," he demonstrates convincingly with a number of solid examples that lowering cholesterol does more harm than cure. High cholesterol does not cause atherosclerosis, and any reputable source will make sure to specify this distinction. Lowering high cholesterol blood levels will make cells more fragile, damage muscle cells and the heart, and reduce the production of our sex hormones. Hence, lowering cholesterol may lead to erectile dysfunction and reduced libido.

In Part VI, "On the Nature of Issues and Disease Related to Physiologic Breakdown," Dr. Dzugan explains why and how certain health issues can be solved by following a physiological approach. If substitution of a certain hormone is necessary, then it should be the correct and biological one. He explains what treatment he suggests for coronary heart disease, macular degeneration, fibromyalgia, and migraine, as well as why.

In Part VII, "On the Nature of Nutrition and Health," he presents his view on how we can get fit and healthy again through life style, diet and exercise. His key message is, "A healthy digestive system is key to a healthy body." He asks the question, "Is fast food by nature and widespread practice unhealthy?" and answers it with "Yes, it is." I have nothing to add in this regard.

This book, written in an entertaining and witty style, is a must for health-conscious people, as are most Americans. Yet, physicians can also learn a lot from Dr. Dzugan's physiological approach in solving health problems. This book serves as an essential guide for anyone who wants to stay healthy and live long.

****

Professor George Birkmayer, MD, PhD.
PhD in Biochemistry, University of Vienna, Austria.
MD from the University of Munich.
Since 1982, Professor of Medical Chemistry, University of Graz, Austria.
Medical Director of the Birkmayer Institute for Parkinson Therapy, Vienna, Austria.
Visiting Professor at the Universities of Beijing, Guangzhou and Xi'An (China).
Fellow of the American College of Nutrition.
President Intl. Academy of Tumour Marker Oncology (IATMO) New York.
Professor George Birkmayer, MD, PhD, discovered the therapeutic effect of NADH (Coenzyme-1) and developed the stabilized orally absorbable form of NADH. Using this formulation, he has treated thousands of patients suffering from Parkinson, Alzheimer, depression, CFS, cancer and diabetes. He is the author of more than 150 scientific publications and member of the editorial board of a number of scientific journals.

INTRODUCTION

Medicine is a complex beast, of that we are all sure. Simply looking at all the vast intricacies of modern medicine can make your head spin. Of course, medicine is a great asset for the sake of the health of billions across the world. It is the way in which we approach treatments of diseases and is how we help people get better.

However, there are chinks in the seemingly impregnable armor of conventional medicine. In certain cases, it has fallen short in its duties to protect and increase health because it focuses not on disease and disorder prevention but on attempts to control the resulting symptoms. Such an approach might not seem like the best, you might say. Those chinks in the armor are there for a reason. Modern medicine stands ready to defend against attack after attack, weakening from the constant battle and failing to prevent casualties.

A different, proactive approach is needed: a physiological approach, to be precise. "Physiology" is a term that references how the body functions under optimal circumstances. A variety of factors influence the slow decrease in adequate body function, which can then lead to a great deal of issues and diseases.

What are the applications of this physiological approach? There are too many to count; the potential scope of its value is huge. Imagine your body working fine. Now, imagine it not working fine. Yeah, it isn't a very pretty picture. As we continue to age, unfortunate issues start to crop up, ranging from heart disease and high cholesterol to declining mental functionality. We become regularly fatigued, our body doesn't seem to want to work like it is supposed to, things that are supposed to stay up would rather stay down, and the list goes on. Fortunately for everyone, the overall health and vitality of our bodies can be restored.

How does the restoration of human physiology work? Well, by restoring its human physiology, of course! This natural approach takes into account a multitude of subsystems that need to be fixed so that the body is rejuvenated to the point of what it was we enjoyed in our twenties. There is no need to dread how the body feels each day in your sixties or seventies. The approach to the restoration of that which makes a fully functioning human work as well as a well-oiled machine comes purely from a natural direction and with no pharmaceutical intervention.

What can be gained from this? Well, it will become clear to you that there's a great deal to be gained. Remember that its applications know no bounds. Recall all the "age-related" diseases that afflict so many people who say it's just because they are getting "old." This common and "natural" affliction does not have to be the case. Age-related diseases and impairments are in large part related to the gradual decline in the body's physiology. By going to town on the cause of the breakdown, rather than trying to fix what keeps being impaired by the breakdown, improvements can be achieved that not only greatly improve health but also the quality of life.

In this narrative, we will be looking at many different issues, all framed with the restoration of physiological function in mind. We will observe how medicine has been shaped into its current form, as well as some of the problems associated with its conventional approach. We shall see where conventional medicine has overwhelming success across a large sector of healthcare, as well as the places in which it could use a hand. We will discuss at length the science behind physiological decline, as well as how it can be restored. We will also look at some of the diseases and issues associated with this breakdown, such as heart disease, high cholesterol, psychological disease, and many other issues that can all be approached in this natural way.

Above all, we want to present as much information as we can in the best way possible so that you can have a better understanding of how your body works and how you can restore your health. As you read, if you have any further questions that weren't particularly answered within the narrative, you can refer to the Dzugan Physiologic website at www.dzlogic.com or call us at 1-866-225-4877.

THE RESTORATION OF THE HUMAN BODY
IN SEVEN PARTS

A doctor teaches his students by dissecting a corpse. Our standards of science have advanced greatly, and thankfully, so have our standards for neck frills and hats.

PART I

On the History of Medicine and the Nature of Disease

What is medicine? Well, the answer to that one is probably quite obvious, isn't it? Medicine is the proverbial art of healing, that oldest of traditions in which individuals, usually doctors who know more than you do, tell you what to do so you can (probably) get better. Although simple in concept, there are so many different phrases thrown around in the air concerning medicine that it can become a bit of a pain to juggle them all and make sense out of all the bedlam.

For example, there is our dear old brother, "conventional medicine," that beautiful majestic beast that holds fast with science, studies, and successes. He is held up as a trusted beacon of "making people feel better" and being an ever-advancing juggernaut by virtue of acting as a cure for innumerable diseases and ailments. Globalization doesn't hurt either. So, conventional medicine is the big boss in the world of the healing arts, and all those "alternative," shady guys can't be trusted, right?

Here is where the door opens and our friend, "the status quo" (the concept, not the well-known band hailing from the United Kingdom) enters, and he says, nay, he yells, "Get these hippies off the doorstep of our majestic palace of conventional medicine, built from years of experience and learning. We need not your powdered keratin from certain odd-toed ungulates or your exotic herbs of horny goats to cure our erectile dysfunction, for we are blessed by the powers that be with the glorious $C_{22}H_{30}N_6O_4S$, as you plebes might know of it, the blue pill!"

With this mighty proclamation, the status quo stands firm, conventional medicine is superior, and all is well in the world. The unwashed masses of "the rest of those guys" are swept away by the power and logic of conventional medicine. After all, the opposite of conventional is unconventional and for good reason! Although the mighty, well-oiled conventional army is fighting the good fight, the unconventional forces are rabble-rousing guerrilla fighters in the bush, and who wants those guys on our side?

Everything surrounding conventional medicine, from the status quo to terminology, the court of public opinion, and patents, all reinforce the fact that being the big boss isn't simply a position that is given. Rather, it is taken by what works and is the most powerful, which also labels it the most useful. Yet, can the unconventional work and be useful and rise in its power? Perhaps we can rewind time and see what has been conventional and unconventional throughout the ages. Maybe by starting from the start, we can figure out where medicine now stands.

Caveman Cures

We begin not in the olden days, but with a detour to our animal friends. What's this, you ask, why in the world are we talking about animals? Well, the thing is that medicine as a concept is not solely the domain of humankind. For example, various monkeys have herbal remedies for relieving menstrual cramps, elephant mothers eat the bark of certain trees to induce labor, and pet house cats sneak out to eat grass when they are not plotting our downfall. There are many more examples, and on top of the ones observed by humans, there are certainly other animal "medical" practices out there. We can now move into more familiar territory.

When we consider the history of human medicine, our collective memories as human beings might likely go immediately back to the Greek pioneers of this very field. Because clearly, every child in Samoa has a rich cultural history passed down by the oral traditions of those crafty Greeks (thanks, globalization). The reason we think of the Greeks is because conventional medicine is also "Western medicine," and as such, we often look to our toga-wearing brothers and sisters as the progenitors of medicine.

As we just said, animals take all kinds of great herbs for all kinds of things. What does that have to do with anything? One would presume that most humans (on average) are smarter than most animals. Just don't say that anywhere a raven can hear you (which is everywhere). Ever since we humans took on the distinction of being the smartest mammals on the block, we did not just magically form our own taxonomic classification with fresh new things and a sudden, exquisite knowledge of medicine. We built it up.

Knowledge about good medicinal herbs was certainly passed down and utilized, by learning through oral traditions. As soon as *Homo neanderthalensis* Bobby took note that a certain plant cured his diarrhea, he certainly passed this key information along to his mammoth-hunting brethren. If he didn't, then he kept the information to seize power and become chief, and we aren't here to judge Bobby's power-hungry ambitions.

In archaeological excavations of early humankind during the periods in which the practice of ceremonial burials is documented, certain key observations are noted regarding the dead. In one particular dig site, dubbed Shanidar Cave, in northern Iraq, the remains conveyed significant information about their owners. One set of remains showed an individual missing a lower arm, with one potential cause being amputation, as well as a severe, crushing blow to the skull.

Looks like Neanderthal Bobby had an accident and perished then? Actually, based on the remains, both of these unfortunate events occurred well before death, and our Neanderthal friend potentially reached his late forties. Although late-forties is an early sendoff in our time, back in the olden days when ol' daddy had to fend off saber-teethed tigers and Austrian barbarians, the forties would be considered as the grandfather age. Bobby was, at this time, telling his Neanderthal grandchildren about how good he had it before he lost part of his arm and had that crushing injury happen to his face, no doubt from those jerk *Homo sapiens* who just moved into the cave just over that hill there.

Another set of remains in the same site shows an individual with advanced osteoarthritis, meaning his people didn't just put him out to pasture when they noticed he wasn't keeping up with the mammoth hunting party. These findings indicate a significant level of care applied to individuals after traumatic injury or debilitating conditions. Significantly, this site is dated between 60,000 to 80,000 BC (radio-carbon dating is a fickle mistress, but what's 20,000 years between old friends?). For those keeping track, this is at least 59,000 years before the Greeks were doing all their fancy Greek things for which we remember them for, and we don't mean the Spartan toga parties. Don't forget, these aren't *Homo sapiens* but rather *Homo neanderthalensis,* our "caveman" cousins.

The most important thing to take away from this is that this site is just one that we have actually found. This was certainly not an isolated incident of altruistic individuals taking care of their sick. Just like courageous, hat-wearing archaeologists are always finding out in movies, there are a lot of things we don't know about. How far back medicine truly goes is a mystery to be sure because, although medicine might have slowly accumulated into a knowledge databank, empathy toward other humans has surely been around for a while, in most cases anyway. Certainly empathy would have made Bobby share the diarrhea cure with his friends (or not, but again, we aren't going to judge because maybe someone said something bad about his mammoth hide yurt into which he had put so much work).

Erudite Egyptians and Persian Physicians

Now that we have covered medicine's prehistoric deep roots, we can move on to those Greeks we mentioned. Well, actually, those philosophers and spreaders of democracy are going to have to get in line again because we can find medicinal use before their time. Let's time travel yet again back to when Egypt had become a unified kingdom around 3150 BCE.

This period was decent bit before well-muscled Spartans (and a couple thousand of those "other" Greeks forgotten by popular lore) held the line at the Battle of Thermopylae. Egypt was a long-standing kingdom of many noteworthy individuals. Therefore, for medicine history purposes, the focus is on one individual: Imhotep.

Today, when many people think of Imhotep, they think of a mighty Egyptian who had an affair with the Pharaoh's concubine, raised the dead, caused plagues, and fought handsome actors in order to control the world. Hollywood might have embellished several key aspects, but it cannot be denied that Imhotep was an extremely intelligent and influential man. On top of building the first true stepped pyramid with uncanny mathematical accuracy (contrary to popular belief, there is more to building a pyramid than putting a bunch of stones on top of each other), he was somewhat of a medicinal wizard, as well.

Writings attributed to Imhotep point to him having a detailed knowledge of disease and cures. Our knee-jerk reaction to hearing of these "cures" might be to snidely think that the best-kept secret in ancient Egyptian "medicine" was to pray to Anubis to not take a patient too soon. Don't judge too soon. Records indicate that Imhotep had what we can call "case studies" for

prospective students that discussed many procedures, such as how to properly heal grievous head injuries that penetrate the brain. That's right. Not only did Imhotep excel at building pyramids and raising the dead, he had a knack for brain surgery, as well. Based on such evidence, from around 2,600 BC, it might even be prudent to say that Imhotep could supplant Hippocrates as the "father of medicine." Does that sound good? If so, watch out because Westernization's status quo will shout at you for disavowing your father of medicine. On the other hand, if you're not ready to let go and embrace Imhotep, then don't worry; we'll yank you out of the status quo soon enough. For the moment, comfort yourself with the fact that Hippocrates still has the distinction of being the "father of Western medicine" because, clearly, Imhotep was a bit south of "West."

Nevertheless, Hippocrates certainly did advance medicinal knowledge. The Greek is so well known in the medical field today that full-fledged doctors still swear the Hippocratic Oath. The entirety of the original is not used now, but its overall ideal of "do no harm" is a concept that is still very strong in this oath. Of course, Hippocrates' medical understandings were not exactly up to par with modern knowledge (hindsight is always 20/20). However, he did establish that diseases have natural origins, and as such, treatments or studies can be made of them. This was an essential idea because it allowed practitioners to treat disease without fearing that Poseidon would drown them in a flood for tampering with his curses. Being unconventional is not blasphemous. Thanks to Hippocrates, the concepts of "modern" medicine really began to take form at this point.

A major idea behind medicine from this period onward was the concept of the four major "humors," which were blood, black bile, yellow bile, and phlegm. They were linked to the seasons and to the "four elements" of air, earth, water, and fire. You can probably see where this is going. "Hah, what outdated and silly notions," you might think. Unfortunately, said silly notions persisted until the 19th century. So, the majority of the history of "conventional" medicine consisted of achieving a balance between the four humors and the four elements, and there is not much humorous about that. If a local physician told us that our touch of the tuberculosis was due to an unbalanced composition between air and water, you might say we would be concerned.

In general, medical knowledge and advancements seem to have been acquired and accomplished in bursts by particularly talented individuals. We can move right on through Medieval medicine by saying, "Boy, are you lucky you weren't sick back then, at least in mainland Europe!" If you were in the "Middle East," Imhotep's old abode, your chances were actually better. Perhaps surprisingly, a lot of good medical knowledge in the Medieval period arose not from Europe but from Arabic doctors, such as Ibn al-Nafis (full name being, of course, Ala-al-din abu Al-Hassan Ali ibn Abi-Hazm al-Qarshi al-Dimashqi, as we're sure everyone knows). He was the first person we know of to describe pulmonary circulation (the novel concept that the heart pumps oxygen-depleted blood to the lungs and receives back oxygenated blood), which he did in the mid-13th century. Another medieval Arabic provider of good medical knowledge is Abu al-Qasim al-Zahrawi, who, circa 1,000 CE, wrote an encyclopedic collection of medical practices and is sometimes referred to as "the father of modern surgery."

Belgian Breakthroughs and English Epidemiologists

Medicine did not progress much further until the beginning of the 16th century when a Flemish doctor, Andreas Vesalius, published a comprehensive book on anatomy. It was called *De humani corporis fabrica libri septem* (otherwise known as *On the fabric of the human body in seven books*, the seven books because, back then, everything was in Latin and you had to make it count). He sought to improve the many Greek errors by drawing illustrations of actual dissections and creating a valuable anatomical map of the human body. Although Vesalius made mistakes in his anatomical comprehension, as well, we can give the guy a break because our ancestors of the 16th century were still grappling with the concept of a heliocentric model of Earthly orbit. Surely, medicine had nowhere to go but up. Well, slowly up, but up somewhat nonetheless.

The 18th century saw major events like the first successful appendectomy (a minor procedure now), and the discovery that citrus fruit cures scurvy (much to the relief of pirates and sailors who no longer had to have bleeding gums). During this time, vaccination procedures began to take root in Europe. Although this is the well-known beginning of the history of vaccination, there are ninth-century-records from India that indicate the procedure (complete with a description of microbe action in theory), but Westernization won't hear any of that. Although microorganisms were "discovered," as in actually observed under the scrutiny of a microscope, by the late 17th century, the theory linking germs to disease didn't get properly established as a widely held "belief" until the later 19th century via the works of Robert Koch and Louis Pasteur. When introduced, this "outlandish" notion was highly controversial in the medical and scientific communities.

As we round the end of the 19th century and go full blast into the 20th, the pieces all start to fall into place and are far too numerous to list. We already skipped over earlier historical examples in the interest of time. After all, you need only a brief overview of the history of medicine to see how conventional medicine evolved. Should you be hankering for some more information about how far medicine has come along, you can always take a gander at the Dzugan Physiologic website on the cover.

We can be very thankful that medicine did evolve so greatly. Imagine if you had to be bled for every ailment or had your foot chopped off by a medieval doctor because that lesion on your toe looks borne of witchcraft. Yeah, those were the good ol' days all right! Now we just have advanced surgical procedures and all the pills we could ever desire.

However, the history of medicine has something very important to teach us. Through that short jaunt through history, remember one thing: Conventional medicine hardly seems conventional in the long run.

For example, the dastardly notion that surgical instruments must be disinfected and hands washed was an unconventional proposition by Joseph Lister that is now an integral part of modern surgical and medical procedures. The unconventional alternative only becomes the conventional norm when enough individuals acknowledge that the practices and treatments are viable and work at a fundamental level. Unfortunately, although conventional modern medicine is a great benefit to humanity and part of the reason as to why we spit in the face of Malthusian population checks, there are certain areas of it that are not utilized to the best extent, that are not based around the core tenets of medicine.

To go fully in depth here, we have to identify the major causes of disease and illness. Before proceeding, we need to clarify the catchall term "disease." For example, both AIDS and depression are diseases. However, it would be more adequate to describe AIDS as an infectious disease and depression as a mental disorder. Only by understanding our enemy, can we fight the enemy, and so on and so forth. We will begin by simplifying all disease as either infectious or non-infectious, and we will further divide the latter into two subcategories—with a special guest star at the end that will lead into the main focus of restorative medicine.

Hey, guy! Is it cool if I hang out here?

Of Vectors and Viruses

Infectious disease is what many of us think of when the word "disease" is mentioned. These diseases are "catchable" and are spread via vectors. A "vector" is an organism that transmits a disease, such as mosquitoes and malaria or people who don't cover their mouths in a crowded elevator when they have a touch of the Spanish Flu because, hey, it's totally not bad manners or a crime against hygiene and mankind to do that. Although it would be nice to think that there is an innumerable host of microscopic organisms out there that want us dead, this isn't really a fair assumption. Actually, that isn't a very nice picture at all. What we can say is that it is all relative. Consider cholera. *Vibrio cholerae* just wants to breed uncontrollably and do what all living organisms want: live and prosper. Unfortunately, to further its ability to live and prosper, cholera has figured out that the side effects of violent diarrhea and vomiting are going to spread more cholera to more people. Cholera by no means wants us to die, it just wants to spread as far as it can. Technically speaking, the most successful infectious microorganism is the one that keeps the host alive as long as possible.

Cholera may not actually ask your permission to "hang out," which is rather annoying. We all know someone like that, don't we? However, all cholera wants to do is stay alive. The only problem is those pesky side effects, the manifestations of the disease that just might cause us to die, which neither cholera nor us want. Even so, cholera goes and ruins it for everyone, wanting too much of a good thing. We all know someone like that, too. Planet Earth is probably saying right now, "Yeah, Mars, I've had this case of the humans for a long time, but the little buggers have really been a pain in the last couple of centuries. This is worse than the time Theia collided with me and formed that jerk, the Moon."

Relativity aside, what we want to do is kill the invaders because we are humans and that's how we take care of business. In the cholera example, we can look at bacteria, with bacteria being one of the four antagonists when speaking about infectious disease. Diseases caused by bacteria includes cholera, typhus, bacterial meningitis, bacterial pneumonia, and the list goes on. The appropriately named antibiotics can kill off bacteria. However, the extremely fast division and growth of bacteria allows for relatively fast evolutionary processes, which in turn, allow them to eventually adapt to antibiotics. Antibiotic-resistant bacteria pose a serious issue because more powerful antibiotics have to be used until, in some cases, they simply stop working. Good news for them; bad news for us. As far as harmful bacteria are concerned, over-the-counter antibiotics are the best things to ever happen to them.

Fungal infections are those caused by fungi. Although we may laugh about athletes foot in the locker room, fungal infections can become a serious matter. Some fungi can cause forms of pneumonia and meningitis, which are a bit rougher than a bad case of athlete's foot. Black mold, other than having a name appropriate for something that lives in a city built of nightmares, grows in damp places and can cause serious respiratory infections. The problem with this one is that said damp places usually happen to be homes in which people breathe in the black mold's mycotoxins (toxins produced via the metabolism of molds). The route of attack against fungi is in the appropriately named antifungal drugs (we are beginning to see a pattern here). Much like bacteria, fungi can become resistant to these drugs, but instead of a good basket of truffles, as everything should result in, it results in a heaping portion of disease that is resistant to drug therapy.

Next, let's clarify parasitic infections. A parasitic relationship is one in which the parasite lives in or with the host in a non-mutual fashion. This is just like the son who is totally going to eventually go back to college to get a degree in communications and will certainly move out when he does so (and he totally won't just stay home to play online games and eat all your food). Not only do these parasitic types not pay the rent, they slowly set the house on fire. There is no mutually beneficial relationship when parasites are involved. In the context of infectious diseases, parasitic infections are those referring to human parasites, such as protozoa and worms. Suffice it to say, the diseases caused by many parasites are pretty disgusting. After all, worms need to stay in the ground and away from our bodies. However, we can mention malaria, which needs no introduction and causes more than half a million deaths per year in the tropics. Although mosquitoes are a vector, the actual cause is the protist that is transferred via saliva during a bite. The treatments for parasites are as varied as the parasites themselves.

The last well-known villain playing a role in our grotesque theatrical show is the virus. If we were still speaking in Medieval European terms, we could call the virus an unholy manifestation of all that is wrong. The virus certainly causes us some unholy confusion because it is not exactly something that we can, with certainty, call a living thing. Although, it replicates and evolves, it lacks cellular structure and reproduces by spontaneous assembly with the host cells without even having the decency to asexually split. It would seem that when life came into being, the virus didn't want to go with the flow and simply said, "Nah, you guys go ahead. I'm gonna go over here and do my own thing." One would imagine this would have barred the virus from all the good parties, which is why it now has a horrific tendency to cause some of the most serious and resilient diseases known to man.

I'll just be over here, ancient and eternal.

Examples of viruses range far and wide. For example, cold sores are considered little more than a nuisance, but the variant of herpes that causes it is quite widespread, and transmission can occur even when the cold sore is not present. It is not very comforting that this variant of herpes infects more people in the world than it doesn't and that it is just content to stay in our bodies until death. AIDS needs no introduction and is caused by HIV. Our yearly friend, influenza, better known as the flu, is also caused by a virus. Furthermore, certain chronic viruses can also cause cancer in infected victims because, clearly, viruses aren't horrifying enough. Primary treatments for viruses include antiviral drugs. Antibiotics do not work despite the popular misconception, and vaccinations are an effective method of preventing viruses, as well.

That sums our brief rundown of infectious diseases. Do keep in mind that the manifestations of infectious diseases result from how microscopic invaders interact with our bodies. For example, our old friend, pneumonia, is the disease associated with inflammation of the lungs followed by coughing, sharp pain in the chest—the works, so to speak. This is the disease. What's the actual cause? It's whatever you want.

Pneumonia can be caused by bacteria, fungi, parasites, and by those unholy manifestations of un-life, viruses. So, let's say you get vaccinated against a type of bacterial pneumonia (you are vaccinated against that particular microbe from causing this particular type of pneumonia), and you are itching for a fight with this disease. Well, you would be winning that particular fight and be impenetrable until a virus infiltrates your body and causes the disease anyway because you are not inoculated against this viral pneumonia. Simply put, the virus caused that pneumonia.

Of Schizophrenia and Scurvy

True to its name, a non-infectious disease is one that does not spread through a vector. Even the aforementioned virus-caused cancer does not fall under the infectious category because the virus can cause cancer, but the cancer is not the infectious disease. So, what about these non-infectious diseases, then?

Well, they are quite the handful. Seeing the extent of infectious disease, we can then throw in all the rest of the players on the island into the category of non-infectious disease. However, first, we must separate the non-infectious sorts into diseases caused by genes and diseases caused by environmental factors.

First of all, diseases caused by malfunctioning genes are more properly called genetic disorders. Although Down syndrome is technically a disease, nobody calls it Down disease.

Down syndrome is caused when there is extra genetic material on the 21st chromosome (a structure of DNA and proteins, of which we have 23 in total). Down syndrome is characterized by various defects, as well as an increased likelihood of having other conditions. Individuals with Down syndrome are at an increased risk of having congenital heart disease, as an example. Another example of a purely genetic disease is cystic fibrosis, an ailment in which multiple organs, specifically the lungs, cannot function properly.

Genetic disease is not solely linked to congenital defects present from day one. These diseases come about from genes passed down from your forebears. In other words, your ancestors having said disease is an expression of the likelihood of the gene "running in the family." There is a wide assortment of genetic diseases acquired through an increased genetic probability of being passed down. For example, if your father had voices in his head telling him to kill Adolf Hitler, we can surmise two things: that the voices were on the right track and that you might wind up with schizophrenia.

The previous mention of congenital heart disease in Down syndrome patients is something that is very important to mention when speaking about non-infectious disease as either genetic or environmental. Congenital heart disease can arise purely from a genetic abnormality, ranging from DNA mutations to chromosomal irregularities. However, congenital heart disease can also occur due to environmental factors, such as if the mother of the fetus partakes in alcohol during pregnancy or if she is afflicted with certain diseases. Even the aforementioned schizophrenia can result from environmental factors.

Now, we will look at environmental disease because, at the end of the day, there is little more to say on genetic diseases other than, "Man, some stuff is going to get messed up that's outside of your control, and then messed-up stuff will happen." The medical field of gene therapy is still in its relative infancy and far from having mass market consumption, but with increased testing and technology, it is certainly promising.

Environmental disease is the impossibly broad definition of diseases caused by the environment. We are not saying that the plants in your local biosphere are out to get you (but some of them might be) but instead are classifying the environmental factors as anything living or nonliving that has an impact on living organisms (a redundant term since all organisms are, by definition, living, and viruses stay well away with their vile sorcery).

Having covered increased genetic probability, let's look at non-genetically influenced schizophrenia as a good example of the variety present in environmental factors. Some studies bear mention in our example here because they clearly reinforce our earlier environmental distinction. "The environment" does not refer to the type of trees and fauna that exist in your neck of the woods or whether you live in a temperate, broadleaf forest biome or a wet, riparian biome. At least, not specifically it doesn't. The environment is the sum of the parts of the location where you live.

Let's say that you are residing in New York City. That means that you currently live in a temperate, broadleaf forest. However, last time we checked, "skyscraper" is not a part of the natural temperate broadleaf forest biome. So, we can easily say that you live in an urban environment. Accordingly, if you grow up in said urban environment, then your risk of acquiring schizophrenia increases a decent amount simply by virtue of growing up in this urban area.[1] To add salt to the wound, it appears that if you are a member of an immigrant ethnic group and not a native born individual living in an area with a low concentration of your ethnic group, then you are at higher risk of schizophrenia down the line.[2-4]

Although the link is tenuous, there is the possibility that cannabis use is associated with increased risks of psychotic disorders and symptoms.[5] However, one link that is certainly not tenuous is that individuals with pre-existing risks of psychosis are more predisposed to the states induced by cannabis use than are healthy control subjects.[6,7] Although these are actual assessment or control studies, there is certainly no end of anecdotal evidence that while some individuals who partake in marijuana fly up high on the back of magical dragons and become unstoppable hunger machines, others succumb to paranoia.

In one fell swoop, we examined several examples of environmental factors, but perhaps we put too much emphasis on the actual environment that a person lives in. In the interest of diversity, we will go over other examples of environmental factors. Earlier on during our brief run-through of the history of medicine, we mentioned scurvy. Although it may be known simply as the bane of pirates, for most of human history, scurvy has actually been a serious concern during ocean expeditions and long winters full of cured meats. What is the environmental factor at work here?

The long voyages or periods that lacked fresh produce necessitated the storage of food that was cured, salted, or in the form of hardtack rations that could probably be used as bricks if the sailors weren't up to eating tooth-breaking, month-old biscuits. Before the link to citrus fruits was established, would the environmental factor causing scurvy be the lack of oranges and lemons? We now know that vitamin C deficiency is at play here, and those fruits simply happened to have a ready supply of it.

Again, we cannot stress enough that environmental factors are part of the "anything goes" category and not just related to deficiencies of something or variables outside of our control. Rampant tobacco-smoking can lead to chronic obstructive pulmonary disease, which is the ever-potent combination of chronic bronchitis and emphysema. The environmental risk at work here is inhalation of tobacco smoke, which is wholly dependent (outside of uncontrollable second hand exposure) on the individual in question. Even then, certain individuals are still more susceptible to this disease due to genetic factors. [8]

Type 2 diabetes has strong environmental components in both obesity and a lack of physical activity. Surely, you might think, that if you simply keep those two at bay, type 2 diabetes will steer clear of you. However, consider an individual who has a genetic defect that hinders physical activity or has a genetic predisposition towards obesity. Let's spice up the mix even more and say that both of those can also be caused in part or in whole by an infectious disease. This is all on top of the known genetic factors at work in acquiring type 2 diabetes (of which about ten percent are known, meaning that 90 percent of the genetic issues influencing risk factors are unknown).[9]

Clearly, there is a lot of interplay between the types of diseases, and many issues can bounce off of each other to create an ultimately more serious condition. In the midst of all this interplay, environmental disease is where we put the bulk of our focus. We want to look at and discuss disease that is caused by **acquired physiologic errors**. "Physiologic" simply refers to a normally functioning and healthy body, and "physiology" is the science behind it.

What diseases do acquired physiologic errors cause? This is going to seem to come out of left field and include a good bunch, so bear with us. Issues such, as heart disease, depression, arthritis, fibromyalgia, migraine, fatigue, atherosclerosis, and cancer can all fall under this category.

An approach of restorative medicine, which is what we will be discussing from this point on, focuses on addressing the breakdowns of optimal body function by optimizing the body's hormones and nutrients and bringing them optimal levels. The body does try to keep in homeostasis (equilibrium), but things are going to breakdown. When the balance and ratios of hormones within the body breaks down, along with a lack of minerals and vitamins, then things will go south real fast.

"Oh boy! Here we go," you might think. "This old boy is talking about curing cancer by keeping my body's 'hormones' in check and making sure I eat my oranges. I'm beginning to suspect he's actually one of those alternative guys he made fun of in the beginning. No doubt that I'll next be advised to buy some crystals that are attuned to my body's electromagnetic output."

This is where our old friend, simplification, hurls a rabbit punch to our necks so that we'll make the necessary distinctions. The statement "this thing in balance will keep that thing from happening" doesn't take into account the staggering complexity of what goes on in our bodies.

Also, at this juncture we would certainly specify that having a fully optimized physiological profile is a part of avoiding certain cancers and, in general, part of an adequate immune response, which is influenced in large part by the hormones that we will be discussing in detail later. However, if Uncle Boris goes playing around the nuclear reactor, then he is going to get cancer no matter how good his testosterone level is because lethal doses of radiation and cellular matter don't like to mingle. Contrary to popular belief, Vodka does not cure radiation poisoning. So let's amend that inclusion of cancer as "cancers that your body is fully capable of keeping at bay with an optimized physiologic profile if everything is in balance and working A-Okay."

One Malaise, One Route of Attack

This restorative approach to medicine is an effective method of treating disease and ailments acquired by physiologic errors because, ultimately, they are the same disease. This obviously seems like a foreign concept from the get-go because conventional medicine creates very clear separations between diseases. How can we imply that something like heart disease is the same as migraines, osteoporosis, or depression? What we are suggesting is that, at a basic level, they are the same because they have the same issue of suboptimal and unbalanced hormones and are affected by the lack of vitamins and minerals.

One might scoff at the notion of vitamins and minerals and perhaps rightfully so—well, that is if we only followed popular notions and misconceptions in our health-related worldview. Let's not forget our friend, scurvy, the vitamin C deficiency. If you are enjoying not having your gums bleed in traditional pirate fashion, you can thank the adequate vitamin C in your diet. Furthermore, adequate iron in your diet helps stave off a

common form of anemia (a condition where your blood does not have enough red blood cells, which most scholars agree is a good thing to have).

Adequate iodine intake helps the thyroid gland function properly, and one of the jobs of the thyroid gland is to manage how sensitive the body is to its own hormones. A lack of iodine in a mother's diet can cause the birth of children who grow up to be mentally and physically retarded without intervention (no intervention being the usual case because if the mother cannot procure adequate iodine in her diet in her environment, then the child will likely experience it, as well). A lack of iodine during infant development can cause mental retardation. Overall, iodine deficiency is by far the most preventable cause of brain damage and mental retardation in the entire world.[10] Next time you're at the local grocery store, make sure to stop by the iodized salt and say thanks because it's been looking out for you (and you thought you knew who your friends were).

We could certainly go further in detail, but for now, we wanted to provide a cursory glance to dispel preconceived notions. "Make sure you get all your vitamins and minerals" is a phrase that has become almost hackneyed and somewhat jokey, something parents might say to their kids perhaps without even enforcing it themselves. We make an effort to eat healthy foods but usually forget the reason healthy food is classified as such. "Healthy" does not just mean a low fat content or that it lacks excessive amounts of sugar. It refers to the food's beneficial vitamins and minerals.

"But surely," you might ask, "even with a basic root cause, wouldn't certain diseases be caused by imbalances in different areas and necessitate a specific treatment approach? Wouldn't heart disease be caused by a certain imbalance and something like depression is caused by another one?"

Yes and no.

Don't take "one treatment approach" at face value or in the conventional sense or it will sound ridiculous. This is because of what we associate with the word "treatment" based on its association with conventional medicine. What sort of treatment do I get if I have high cholesterol? You take this pill. What sort of treatment do I get when I have depression? You take this other pill. What treatment do I get if I have type 2 diabetes? You take this insulin, you watch your blood sugar, you make sure to exercise, and in general, you avoid behavior that can exacerbate your condition.

Now, we are getting somewhere.

A lot of conventional treatment operates on a 1:1 basis, in which you have one condition and you take one thing from the pharmacy for it. Meanwhile, optimal human physiologic function has an extremely intricate network of links and dependencies that forces anyone who is trying to optimize it to look at the picture as a whole and not just at the symptoms here and there. When we speak of a restorative medicinal approach to the restoration of physiologic function, we throw the 1:1 approach out the window.

Instead, all factors have to be considered. For example, *this* is low and unbalanced. We ask the following questions: What do we have to do to increase that level? What else will this increased level impact? How will this increase benefit another problem in the body? How will the other thing that we are already trying to improve affect the efficiency of this increase? Ultimately, it is most certainly a "one" treatment approach. It just so happens that said treatment seeks to cover every nook and cranny within the body's complex physiologic functionality.

So, what about all this hormone stuff we are talking about? We will address why they are so important, and even sneak in a guest appearance by "big daddy cholesterol." To vividly paint the picture for you, we will discuss the diseases and conditions that arise from the breakdown of physiological function. We will certainly also look at the unfortunate reason these imbalances happen, as well where we can introduce our own approach to correcting these issues.

The ultimate goal here is, first and foremost, the dissemination of information so that you can better understand how your own body works and how complex interaction can be understood and utilized to improve your function. There's nothing so influential and motivating as thoroughly understood new knowledge. However, before we pass out the good stuff, we will first discuss the pitfalls of conventional medicine. *(Insert dramatic fanfare here.)*

Much like Saint George slaying the dragon, conventional medicine has taken out a lot of baddies. Unfortunately, a village or two might have been burned along the way.

PART II

On the Pitfalls of Conventional Medicine

No, wait! It's okay! No need to pull out your tinfoil hats and divining rods, for we haven't gone off the deep end. When we go and say something like "On the Pitfalls of Conventional Medicine," we are going to make certain assuring distinctions. We would not use a dense blanket statement, such as, "Man, that there conventional medicine is all goofed up." No, instead we are going to focus on which parts of conventional medicine under which conditions have the aforementioned pitfalls.

Conventional medicine as a whole is an amazing machine. We have eradicated the likes of polio and smallpox. We have turned diabetes from an extremely premature death sentence into a manageable disease. Millions of infants live today when just more than a century ago they would have been dead before their first day. We are even starting to give HIV a run for its money.

Now, if you go on a whimsical safari to sub-Saharan Africa to see some lions and giraffes and just happen to acquire Ebola, then several things are going to happen. First of all, no matter how good your hormones are and how balanced your body physiology is, Ebola doesn't play around. Now, certainly, if your body physiology is optimized and your internal systems are rearing up and good to go, you could well be amongst the potential ten percent of people who don't die of untreated Ebola.[1] However, with 9:1 odds even before we consider the likelihood of your optimal physiology, our money is going to be on Ebola.

Secondly, not wanting to chance those awful odds, you will be whisked away to a quarantined Ebola ward, set up with emergency protocols in mind, in which you have a 32 percent chance of survival. Although that might not sound like a reassuring number, we can thank conventional modern medicine it's as high as it is. Modern medicine has established the protocols, medication, and necessary research to fight whatever the microscopic world throws at us, even to counteract the brutal damage such diseases can sometimes cause.

So, we have established that conventional medicine, at its core and through many points of its activity and healing methodology, is a very great thing. Generally, it keeps us living longer (we will get right on that in a bit) and just makes things better for us all around.

Now we are going to hit upon the lackluster part.

The problem with the current conventional medical model is that it does not focus on the actual root cause of many diseases and health conditions, but instead goes after the symptoms.

This is where we have to get technical and break it down. First of all, you must note the use of the word "many" in that statement above. It by no means says anything about "all." Let's say that a favored co-worker is trying to be funny and decides to send you an envelope filled with flour. You, being a culinary-challenged individual, believe it not to be the potential gateway to unimaginable gastronomic delicacies, but rather a heaping portion of anthrax spores. You run to the hospital to be checked out and are given a clean bill of health while your co-worker is taken away to be water boarded in the defense of democracy. That'll teach him.

Suppose that you actually did contract anthrax, and *Bacillus anthracis* has gained a foothold in your body. What is going to happen if you rush in for treatment? An extremely potent dose of antibiotics will be put in your body, both intravenously and orally. This treatment regimen will greatly increase your chance of survival because this matchup, antibiotics versus the bacteria, is going after the root cause of the disease by fixing the issue that is causing it.

This perfectly demonstrates where the fruits of our scientific research on antibiotics and our work in epidemiology combine together to identify the root cause of the disease and to focus on eliminating it to fix the problem. Hold on, you might think, but this is related to infectious disease transferred by pathogenic action. What about the diseases related to the breakdown of physiologic function that were mentioned earlier, the kinds that are the non-infectious, environmental sort?

This is an excellent observation, and we commend you. We didn't just put it in your head because we wrote it (why, the very notion!). We want you to think critically and to play the devil's advocate. If you want, you can go practice by advocating for the equal rights of viruses.

What we have to do is shift our *specific* definition of disease. We already covered all those things that can cause coughs, involuntary body effluences, and oozing sores. From this point hence, whenever we refer to disease, we are referring to our particular subset, the familiar neck of the woods that is solely inhabited by diseases that result from bodies that don't work properly due to the breakdown of physiologic function. This precise corner of the woods is from where we will launch our skirmishes against popular concepts and standards regarding the current "treatment" of diseases in our medical system.

Heart Disease and Inadequate Mammoth Hunters

In 2011, the typical family of four in the United States spent $19,393 for healthcare. You might be pensively nodding your head in agreement, perhaps dropping a curse here and there about the "establishment." As with all numbers, relativity helps comprehension. After all, we can hear about the Milky Way galaxy being 100,000 light years across all day long, but until we realize the distance from the Earth to the Sun is only 15.813×10^{-6} light years (it takes sunlight a little over eight minutes to reach the Earth), it doesn't mean much. Back to our more worldly concerns of paying the doctor bills, we can look at 2009 and see that this same cost was $16,771. Meanwhile, those upstart youngsters in 2003 were enjoying a cost of $10,168.[2]

You might wonder what this has to do with our particular target diseases. After all, one does not simply walk into Congress and lower health care costs. This is not the point of this data here. We listed these values because a staggering percentage of that money goes toward the treatment of preventable disease, specifically non-infectious disease (so we aren't bringing vaccines and anti-pathogens into this equation). In fact, coronary heart disease is the leading killer in the developed world.[3-5]

In regards to coronary heart disease, a prolific number of studies have been conducted on this topic, and there are certain variables that remain constant. One specific post-analysis of one particularly large study showed what variables mitigated risk and what variables increased risk. In this analysis, mild to moderate work related to physical activity decreased the risk of myocardial infarction (death of heart cells due to interruption of blood supply), while owning a car and television increased the risk.[6]

Now, don't go throwing out the Toshiba and selling the Toyota just yet. Let's not forget our environmental catchall factors. Owning either of those items simply promotes sedentary behavior, and thus, increases the risk. You can probably see where this is going. If a person performs both regular physical activity and doesn't own a car or television, then he is less likely to be obese (because he is working very hard to afford a car and television).

This large study was large indeed. It tracked 15,152 cases with 14,820 controls across 52 countries on every inhabited continent (Antarctica always gets left out because everyone gives her the cold shoulder). The risk factors for myocardial infarctions in this study were established as abnormal lipids (which include fats and triglycerides), smoking, hypertension (high blood pressure), diabetes, obesity, psychosocial factors (we're looking at you, stress), consumption of fruits and vegetables, consumption of alcohol, and physical activity.[7]

As you can see, these factors are of the preventable variety. Putting out the smuggled Cuban cigar, hitting the gym, not being mistaken for the mall Santa or Mrs. Claus during Christmas time, and drinking less alcohol can give you much better odds. It seems that the developed countries have indeed developed more ways in which to not move around, as well as how to add another flour and cornmeal layer to that fried chicken. The number one killer has never tasted so good. Although we're on the subject of fried fowl, obesity is not only a high risk factor for coronary heart disease but also a big risk . . . period. Much like heart disease, obesity is one of the leading causes of preventable death.[8] In fact, we can quickly deconstruct links to obesity and its role in myocardial infarction as per most of the risk factors that were mentioned.

Here is a list of those factors that determine risk and how obesity is linked to them:

- ❖ High blood pressure—there is a large association between obesity and elevated blood pressure.[9]
- ❖ Diabetes—obese individuals are at a high risk of acquiring type 2 diabetes.[10]
- ❖ Obesity—well, we certainly worked ourselves into a corner with this one.
- ❖ Psychosocial factors—this one is much more variable. In the not so distant past and in various cultures even today, obesity was and is associated with wealth because only a wealthy individual could attain the excess calories, in the form of abundant food and livestock, needed to become and remain obese. In the present day, in the Western world, bacon sandwiches as far as the eye can see are available to the masses, and obesity is generally seen as a stigma. Being obese in a culture that is telling you not to be obese can cause extra stress for the individual.
- ❖ Consuming fruits and vegetables (eating healthy)—who in the world needs to eat healthy when we have double-fried chicken and bacon sandwiches? Besides, pizza has olives on it (but we usually switch those out for extra Canadian bacon). At least it still has tomato sauce. That makes it healthy, right?

❖ Physical activity—while physical activity becomes more and more difficult the more obese one becomes, logic would dictate that perhaps it would be not a bad idea to not let it get that far in the first place. Word on the grapevine is that there is this fad going around called "ambulation," and supposedly, all you have to do is get up and go somewhere. The world certainly is full of silly ideas.

❖ Alcohol Consumption—this link is more tenuous because it certainly isn't 1:1. However, one simply has to think back to the time when Big Jim and the boys are swigging back their 20th brew at the Cotton Fair to remember that basic alcohol consumption includes a lot of empty calories, promoting an entire industry of watered-down beer and elastic waistband manufacturing. Being obese certainly doesn't necessarily make an individual drink, but the drinking itself can plant the seed for obesity in the first place, as well as increasing its severity. It certainly doesn't help that this fermented ambrosia can be addictive.

The only others left on the list are smoking and lipids. Smoking is smoking and, despite the big warnings on the side of cigarette packets and the billboard extinction of beloved, manly, chain-smoking cowboys, is still an addiction of about 21 percent of Americans.[11] Supposedly, lipids include that international felon, cholesterol, but we're going to go into further detail about that later because it covers a very fair portion of coronary heart disease's main co-conspirator—atherosclerosis. Atherosclerotic plaque thickens artery walls by building up upon them, and a component of this plaque is cholesterol. That discussion will naturally include the role of restorative medicine regarding this condition.

On the subject of obesity in the United States, more than one-third (35.7 percent) of adults and 17 percent of children and adolescents are obese. If we consider a state-by-state analysis, data from 2010 shows that not a single state has and obesity rate less than 20 percent. If you traveled across the United States, at the very least, about 21 out of every 100 people (such as in Colorado) you meet will be obese, and in some states this number is as high as 34 out of every 100 people (Mississippi).[12] The "thinnest" state's population has an obesity rate higher than one out of five. We must also keep in mind that obese is obese. If an individual falls into the standard classification of being just "slightly overweight," then they do not factor into those numbers. Our old friend, Caveman Bobby, would probably have some words to say about the dangers and futility of mammoth hunting while having a Body Mass Index (BMI) greater than 30. He might also point out that BMI is a very flawed sort of measurement, but that is neither here nor there.

With some knowledge behind our belt about this particular disease, let's consider how the mainstream conventional medical approach would work, it being a system of reactions in this case as opposed to a system focusing on prevention. Coronary artery bypass surgery is a technique of vein and artery grafting that improves blood circulation to the heart muscle with a potential reduction of the risk of death from coronary heart disease. However, although the benefit of performing this procedure on someone who is actually having a heart attack is known, the benefit for individuals with stable conditions has not been established.

One particular study, conducted over five years, observed patients with coronary heart disease, who were split into two major groups. One group was treated with medical therapy alone while the other was also treated with the bypass procedure. There was no observable difference in regards to total death within the two groups. However, the group that had the procedure did have lower rates of death specifically from cardiovascular causes.[13]

So, who won? Although, the second group did have less incidence of death from the targeted cause, the overall amount of death was not so distinguishable. Dead is dead, as the saying goes. This is something we will be looking at in other instances as another potential pitfall of the conventional approach. A population might be targeted with a specific treatment for a specific condition and not die from that condition, which is good for that population. Still, when the number of deaths within that population increases to as much as it is from other causes or even to a higher rate while undergoing the treatment, the novelty of not dying from the first one quickly wears off.

Another player in the reactive conventional treatment game for coronary heart disease is angioplasty. This procedure involves threading a deflated balloon towards an atherosclerotic deposit and then inflating it, crushing the buildup to improve blood flow. A small tube called a "stent" may be placed in this location to ensure that it stays open. Both this procedure and the bypass can improve chest pain.[14] Unfortunately, it does not increase life span past what can be achieved with therapy nor does it decrease the chance of having a heart attack.[15] Furthermore, there is also the slight chance of the usual surgical complications, heart attack being one of them. Death isn't funny, but it sure can be ironic. At least, if none of the other potential pitfalls brings us down, we can tell our friends and loved ones about that one time when "that doctor totally inflated a balloon in my artery."

In 2006 alone, 1.3 million coronary angioplasty procedures were performed with an average cost of about 48,000 dollars each. There were also 448,000 coronary bypass surgeries at almost 100,000 dollars each. Together, these two operations totaled a bit more than 100 billion dollars in medical costs.[16] The main issue here is that surgical intervention is a high-cost, end-of the-line procedure. If even some of these funds from insurance companies, both public and private, were funneled more into preventative and restorative measures, then the overall costs would go down. Making sure that we turn off the stove before we go out and checking for electrical wiring faults is a whole lot cheaper (or free, as the case may be), than having the house catch on fire and burn to the ground. Insurance can buy us a new house, but it won't buy us a second life.

Fries versus Fiber

So, what about nutrition and healthy eating anyway? Doctors tell us to eat healthy. Is this factor really one of the pitfalls of conventionally medicine? Well, since many of us go to the doctor to pilfer their minds of sound advice in all realms anatomical, one would expect that they have a wealth of advice to offer regarding good eating guidelines. Unfortunately, although medical school is quite a long ordeal, part of said long ordeal doesn't really involve learning about proper nutrition.

A 2007 study of 106 medical schools showed that only 30 percent of them required students to take a separate nutrition course. The average amount of hours received of nutritional education (over the entirety of their school term) was 23.9 with the actual overall hours ranging from two to 70. In other words, some students got 70 hours of nutritional education, but many more got as little as two, bringing that average down quite a bit.[17] Suffice it to say, it doesn't appear that getting your fiber in and making sure to eat those leafy greens is first priority at the endurance ordeal that we call medical school.

Yet, you might say, "Who cares? I hear 'doctor,' I think of surgery and medication." The first is accurate, because although a doctor is not always a surgeon, a surgeon is always a doctor (or at least one would hope). The second is perhaps an unfortunate association. It is true, though, that a huge part of a doctor's training goes into learning how to cut someone open, not in an effort to butcher but in an effort to save, and another huge part into learning the pathways of disease and what medication can be used to help. After all, "medication" is the blanket term for anything that is used to help sick people get better, which would include vitally important items like antibiotics and anti-viral drugs.

However, let's back up and look at the disease that can be caused by improper diet. Obesity and not eating well leads into hypertension, type 2 diabetes, coronary heart disease, and more. Let's not forget that some of those are leading killers. Now, many would say that preventing death from disease is high up on the list of priorities for the medical profession. Thus, although we depend on doctors to help improve our health, we have a high probability of seeing a doctor who has little to no true education about nutrition despite their vast knowledge of their field.

So, whom can we turn to for nutritional advice? Grandma keeps telling us to eat our beets in order to not wind up like Grandpa during the Great War, but we're not all that sure that's enough. Some health magazines and books have recipes, but their overall eating guidelines are often scant, not to mention the fact that the source is in question because journalists aren't exactly high up on the list of people we wish to turn to for health advice. Let's not forget fad diets because what can go wrong from forty-eight hours of juice drinking and fasting?

There are, of course, individuals who may even call their own profession "nutritionist," but that can be a touch sketchy. Many countries have no regulations (or regulations that vary by state or province) whatsoever on who can call themselves a nutritionist, and they lack a system of pre-requisites and standardized practices. Although one nutritionist may have a vast background of encyclopedic knowledge and sound advice about many food types that is backed up by training from an accredited source, another nutritionist might tell you to eat barley for a week straight because "It's totally good for you, man." In this case, the lowest common denominator brings everybody down, and many individuals may likely go to nutritionists who are just a step above "hedge wizard" in the category of "helpful" professions.

Although, if that hedge wizard can make potions for weight loss, then clearly he would be the better choice.

Although the nutritional advice and hedge wizard field is highly likely to improve since preventable disease keeps killing, to some it might not be the best consolation. After all, we go to the doctor to cut us open and graft extra tissue to our hearts to extend our life expectancy. So, we would expect that same doctor to be able to explain to us about eating right ten years prior in order to avoid that operation in the first place. Clearly, the cause of not eating right and the resulting symptoms necessitating the surgery both apply to the disease, and "D" is for disease, but also for doctor.

Jerky Knees and Potent Prescriptions

Ah, meds. As a consumer society, we love us some drugs, as they say in the vernacular. Why, there are pills for everything you could ever dream of! There are diet pills that most certainly make us feel like trans-dimensional warriors separated from our bodies to no longer feel hunger or emotion, and we certainly are not describing that from any personal experience. If we feel blue, are in a blue house, and everyone around is blue, there are certainly pills to add additional colors to our world so that we can go out and perhaps go to Paris to see the Eiffel Tower like that time in 1965. There are even pills that help us apprehend that international fugitive, cholesterol. Let's say we want to go out on the town and party (and by party, we mean ordering the seven-layer nachos filled with strata upon strata of melted cheese and potent peppers). We have meds to help us weather the initial digestive onslaught and the inevitable cataclysm of purging fire that follows the next morning as sure as the sun rises in the east.

The problem with such drugs, be they prescription or over the counter, is that they are not treating the base cause, the disease, but are instead trying to treat the symptoms. Let's say a dam has a crack in it and is slowly flooding the valley. Engineers come up with the brilliant plan of putting in great big pumps into the valley to suck all the water up while releasing heavy smoke into the air from the process, and everyone applauds this move as a wise decision. You might say that this sounds like it makes no sense and is perhaps even borderline illogical. What "logic" is to be had here? Well, we get those engineers, we give them some steel and cement, and we get those boys to fix the dam. It's simple and good.

Despite the nonsensical nature of this example, it can be applied directly to many popular drug treatments today. We take a quick look at the underlying causes of disease, then say, "Ha, screw that," and then go and start treating the symptoms. How is treatment accomplished? It's done in the simplest way possible: a trip to the pharmacy for a pill bottle. The pill is taken to treat the symptom, to remove the flooding waters. The symptom isn't getting better, or at least not for long, because the cause of the symptom is not being addressed; the crack in the dam is still there. There is even likely to be side effects, the heavy smoke in the air.

Instead of fixing our dams, we pollute the air and pump out the water, until that original crack grows big enough and the entire thing breaks and floods the valley even more. This is of course considering we don't choke on the smoke first. When do we get to breathe in relief, to feel refreshed after our restored health?

To see the prevalence of prescription drugs, one only needs to turn on the television and wait for a commercial break. The game is won as soon as an advertisement concerning prescription drugs comes on. We would not advise anyone to use this as the basis of a drinking game, however, because by the second hour, someone just might black out and suffer from cirrhosis.

Okay, so they didn't fix the dam, and now we're choking on smoke. What's next? Next, you get the application of drugs for what are ultimately side effects. This is little more than a "band-aid" effect. Ah, yes, a simple band-aid. That makes sense. You might wonder why we went with the dam analogy instead of the simple band-aid one since you are likely to be wearing one right now if you didn't take our earlier advice about not saying that humans are the smartest when ravens are nearby. We didn't go for that because a band-aid is actually useful. The convenient adhesive strip keeps in place the pad that seals out germs and dirt, the presence of which might prolong wound-healing or even make it infected and worse. Still, when used properly, the band-aid is useful. It might even have anti-bacterial properties. The point is that it accelerates the wound-healing process. To call symptom-treating drug use a band-aid is to give band-aids a bad reputation. This sort of drug application can be likened to a band-aid, all right, but it would be a band-aid that looks exactly like your skin, one that covers up the wound, so as not to notice the underlying issue, and never allows any actual healing to take place while increasing your risk of cancer on the side.

We can take a brief look at statin drugs as an example of our dam scenario, particularly because it works so well. For those unfamiliar with the term "statin," it is simply a reference to the most popular type of cholesterol-lowering drugs. All statins are cholesterol-lowering drugs, but not all cholesterol-lowering drugs are statins. Other cholesterol-lowering drugs include selective cholesterol inhibitors, bile acid sequestrates, and fibrates. The names alone show that there is more than one way reduce cholesterol, but here we focus on statins because of the way they work.

Statin drugs hold the distinction of being the most powerful boys on the block, both in terms of the power of their effects and their revenue. In fact, cholesterol-lowering drugs are generally the cream of the crop when it comes to bringing in the bank. We could have sworn that the main purpose of drugs was supposed to be something else, but we can't quite place our fingers on it. Lipitor®, a cholesterol-lowering drug, was already the best-selling pharmaceutical drug in 2003 back when it was still under patent.

So, what kind of side effects are we talking about here from statin medications? You know, the usual. One that is always good to talk about is *myopathy*. Myopathy simply means muscle disease in Greek (does nobody in the medical community speak English?) and can be described as muscle weakness caused by the faulty function of muscle fibers. Well, that sounds pretty mild, if all we have to worry about is maybe not being able to lift some weights here and there and maybe having a sore arm. The problem here is that the ol' heart is just a big muscle, and a pretty important one at that. This myopathy can affect the pumping function of the heart, a function some would say is best left unaffected.[18]

From myopathy, we can piggyback onto another more serious side effect called *rhabdomyolysis*. Rhabdomyolysis is the rapid breakdown of skeletal muscle cells, which can lead to serious issues. "Skeletal muscle" is the term for the muscle used to move the skeleton, which is an odd way of phrasing all the muscles that we use for locomotion. The biceps and triceps that you are using to hold up this book (or e-reader, you dastardly technophile) are an example of skeletal muscle. We don't want to go too deep into the scientific details of skeletal muscle breakdown and how it leads to dangerous complications, but suffice to say that a bunch of stuff comes out that is not meant to that begins to cause some damage. Are statin drugs the only way to potentially get rhabdomyolysis? Certainly not!

There is a plethora of things just waiting out there for the opportunity to damage your skeletal muscle. Some violent examples that come to mind are getting struck by lightning or receiving a crushing injury from the likes of a car accident. Other examples include heatstroke and viral infections. Although the common reactions to rhabdomyolysis include nuisances like muscle pain, weakness, confusion, and nausea, complications can arise that include the likes of an inflamed liver, an irregular heartbeat, and cardiac arrest. Furthermore, acute renal failure is a very dangerous complication that happens in 15 percent of individuals with rhabdomyolysis.[19] This is simply another term for acute kidney failure, which has a high incidence of mortality (the overall measure of deaths in a population). We can make do without one kidney, but when both lefty and righty are taken out, the prognosis quickly becomes rather bleak.

One particular statin drug, Baycol®, was pulled from the worldwide market in 2001 because the incidence of fatal cases of rhabdomyolysis was between 16 and 80 times greater than with other statin drugs.[20] Based on all this data, we can make some tentative statements. Now, we're not going to say that taking statin drugs is the same as getting struck by lightning because that isn't a fair comparison. We're just going to note the fact that what can happen to your skeletal muscle system when you get struck by an exceptionally large bolt of electricity hotter than the surface of the sun can also potentially happen if you take an easy-to-swallow pill in order to manage your cholesterol. We always try to be optimistic; there aren't many links present between manifestations of the rage of Zeus and medical treatment.

At this point, the side effects are going to keep rolling in, and so we'll make a quick list of some others for easy perusal:

❖ Statin therapy can be a cause of cognitive impairment (I can't think, good doctor!), dementia (who bought me these awful pants and what year is it?), memory loss (I really hope I'm not a government assassin because I honestly can't remember!), and peripheral neuropathy (my arm won't stop twitching and my nerves are hurting something fierce!).[21-25]

❖ There have been documented cases of lupus-like conditions, inflammation of the lungs and chest, and joint pain without swelling.[26] If there is one type of condition that an individual likely does not want to have, it would certainly be one that is lupus-like.

❖ The occurrence of side effects has been observed to be as high as 73.6 percent and 74.9 percent for certain statin drugs.[27]

❖ Although statin drugs decrease death from heart disease by 15 percent, this is offset by increased deaths from cancers, gallbladder disease, and injuries.[28] As always, when we deal with an end result of death in cases and studies such as these, it tends to overshadow everything else. If 20,000 people were on statin drugs and less died from heart disease but the overall number of coffins filled was the same, then they might not tend to care about how they died. Death is a serious "condition," and the end-result does not become milder for the one experiencing it just because of how it happened.

❖ Higher incidences of cancer in groups using cholesterol-lowering drugs has been noted, specifically in regards to gastrointestinal cancer.[29]

❖ Advertisements imply that a multitude of older individuals are taking cholesterol-lowering drugs while going on exciting mountain-biking expeditions and kayaking trips, happy as can be. Well, one would assume that if they were having such a great time they'd just keep taking cholesterol-lowering drugs for a while. After all, those mountains aren't going to bike themselves. Studies show instances in which 60 percent of users discontinued their medication over a period of 12 months, and only one-third of people on a lipid-lowering regimen finish it.[30,31] Maybe those mountains are going to have to wait after all.

Certainly none of these side effects are pleasant, hence their label. So, let's tie this in with our previous issue: cost and convenience. The best approach to medicine is certainly not looking through the green tint of money and how it is impacted. However, the exchange of goods and services does in fact run on money in the modern world. We can't give our doctors some apples in a barter exchange for a colonoscopy because that isn't how it works anymore and we would certainly be sad about the amount of apples we would have to give up anyway. That's not to mention the fact that we would be setting ourselves up for a fall by getting rid of all those apples since they contain agents that can prevent colorectal cancer.[32]

Freedom Isn't Free (Neither is Healthcare)

Let's consider cost. We've already noted how expensive angioplasties and coronary bypass procedures are each year, as well as the vast amount of people who get them. Although the cost of each operation may seem excessive and perhaps even astronomical (or outright impossible for people who can't afford them), we must always keep in mind that surgery has an extremely large amount of factors that go into the cost. It is easy to brush off that cost as going towards our local doctor's "Ferrari Fund," but obviously (hopefully obviously), this is far from the truth. The equipment, the medication, the possibly multiple doctors and the requisite multiple nurses, the building the operation is performed in . . . Well, we could keep going for a while. All these factors can increase the cost by quite a bit because they aren't exactly cheap. We are certain most would agree that this system is still better than your doctor getting you drunk and cutting you open on that bit of comfortable grass in the nearby meadow.

Moving away from the costs to the operators, we mustn't forget the people going under the knife. Even though they usually pay a monthly insurance fee, not all policies are created equal and the patient might pay for the procedure from everyone's favorite money source: out-of-pocket. Depending on the surgery, the patient might have to stay in the hospital for post-operative recovery, and hospital room stays don't exactly price themselves according to roadside motel nightly rates.

Last, we can never forget about the government and our most beloved friends, the insurance companies. On an individual basis, we might be unhappy with paying the health insurance each month, but we have to consider how the system works. Naturally, part of the cost is devoted solely to profit (as in any business anywhere), but even so, the insurance company isn't exactly just squirreling away mountains of cash all the way to the bank.

Let's say that the cost of an operation is a whopping 90,000 dollars and is completely covered for the individual who is using the insurance. Now let's say that 900 people are paying 100 dollars a month for insurance. Obviously, this example is greatly simplified in the interest of easy mathematics because we want to leave the calculus to the engineers working on alternative energy sources. For the insurance company to cover this operation expense, it would use the monetary equivalent of 900 monthly payments from a group of people at a certain level of insurance. To put it another way, it would use the same amount of money that an individual paying the 100 dollar monthly rate would have paid over the course of 75 years.

Keeping operator costs, your costs, and your insurance company's costs in mind, let's now look at how the government plays into this. Of course, this depends entirely on your country. In the United States, our default example, the government has Medicare, which covers about 48 million people out of the 313 million people in the latest total population figures. This government-run insurance system covers slightly less than 50 percent of all costs for individuals who have it. We would obviously modify this value greatly for countries that have a much more robust or all-inclusive public health system. The point is that such government programs are funded through taxes, which are paid by citizens.

Ultimately, in either case, the people are paying for their health care. So, what happens when, instead of cheaper preventative measures, the number of surgeries and complicated interventions slowly keeps rising? The overall cost to the people, regardless of private or public insurance, will go up. One thing to remember is that people can grumble a good bit about paying for health insurance, but they are going to complain even more about paying higher taxes.

Instead of the most expensive game of "pick your poison' ever, perhaps some common sense needs to be injected into the modern medical system. Common sense ties in with convenience. It is much more convenient to take some lighter preventative measures instead of being cut open by a surgeon down the line. The benefits of fewer surgeries and complicated medical interventions would filter down to the people paying for these things in the first place, and everyone would function a little bit better. There is even the potential for the coverage of more issues and treatments through insurance, because so much money would no longer be thrown into the whirlpool of preventable disease management and complex intervention.

The long and short all of this is that a bigger focus on a preventative medical approach is ultimately the superior choice when it comes to addressing disease. Spending would be decreased across the board, from the individual at the bottom of the contributory scale (which interestingly enough is also the part of the scale that is affected the most) to the very top at the corporate and government levels. The possibility of extending government insurance to more people or decreasing the cost of private insurance could also open up the door to the uninsured. A recent study showed that up to 45,000 working-age Americans die due to being uninsured unlike their privately insured counterparts. Ideally, such a number would not exist anymore because insurance would be more affordable to the people in question or the government would be able to further extend its help.[33]

Most importantly, such an approach to medicine has the potential to greatly increase the quality of life for all those involved. We have previously discussed certain suboptimal treatment procedures associated with conventional medicine and preventable disease, but other than the controllable environmental risk factors that were covered, there hasn't been much elucidation about alternative therapies. Well, we're about to fix that by first introducing you to the key players in the hormone game, a cut-throat affair in which some will overtake you by strength while others will make you bleed regularly. Don't worry; we'll make sure you make it out of there. We'll even show you how to win.

Although Heracles gets the *lion's share* of credit for his heroic exploits, much of his success can be attributed to what must have been a god-like amount of testosterone. Ancient Greek secrets and all that . . .

PART III

On the Nature and Effects of Hormones

So, what's all this about hormones? We know, you keep asking, and we keep delaying the answer by delving into the other parts that make up the whole of the picture of the restoration of your health. Well, now we shall indulge your request. Hormones: We all have them and know that those darn teenagers have perhaps too many of them, but we as a society have been conditioned with both apathy and mistrust in regards to these vital substances.

If hormones are as important as we are implying, the full scope of importance being revealed in this chapter, then you may ask why we still suffer from those preventable diseases. If hormones are so powerful in relation to our health, then why don't they counteract our smoking, our obesity, or our diabetes? Hormones already do their job all too well. So, what's the problem?

Time is the problem. Well, not specifically time because, although the understanding of time may help us go into the far future in order to flee from communist-inspired underground dwelling creatures, it won't stop our hormones from going down. We are talking about time in the sense that it passes, and while time passes, we are hopefully alive to see it pass, and thus, we age.

Think back to that old Chevy (or Peugeot, if you are so inclined and perhaps are also French) you have sitting out in the driveway. Always you had thought, 'Man, I had so much fun on that old boy, I'm definitely going to take care of it and polish it up, and I'll definitely fix up the old engine, make her purr like a kitten hittin' 100 down the freeway.' Then, perhaps the Chevy is still sitting out there in disrepair. Maybe you've been too busy, or maybe your wife thinks that Chevy restoration money is better spent on your kid's college education. Perhaps it's in the garage or has a tarp over it. Regardless of where it is, if you aren't keeping up with it and making sure all the internal systems are in working order and that the paint is still as good as that time you went down to the levy, then that Chevy isn't exactly going to run well nowadays.

The human body is much like an automobile. In the prime of its existence, both the car and yourself will have a ball, going fast and hauling lumber for your next great construction project. However, much like that old Chevy, if the human body isn't given proper care, it will go into decline. Unfortunately, although we can tune up the old car and make it run "good as new," the situation is a bit more difficult on the biological side.

We humans, as organisms, age, and when we age, our overall functionality begins to decline. Unfortunately, we aren't possibly immortal like lobsters may be (a thought to keep in mind next time you go out for seafood).[1] We are also not highly resistant to extreme heat, cannot laugh in the face of overwhelming radiation, sneer at atmospheric pressure higher than the depths of the ocean, or survive in outer space like the water bears (tardigrades). No, we are just humans, and even though we may have invented majestic, individually sealed snack cakes, we nonetheless perish due to our mortality.

Did you hear the one about humans trying to live in outer space? Hah, how droll!

Before we do ultimately perish, we go through stages of life. Before our teens, we develop quickly and absorb information like a sponge. Time moves slowly because we haven't yet lived long enough to see how fast it moves in comparison to the span of our lives, and we have boundless energy with which to run around on grand adventures inside haunted mansions. When the teenage years hit, puberty came at us like the world champion at the demolition derby. Those hormones that we always blame for the behavior of teenagers is simply a large spurt of production tying into the transition to adulthood, which some individuals find hard to cope with, the ungrateful little curs.

Next, comes the roaring twenties. This decade of life is when hormone production in the human lifespan is at its peak. During the inordinate amount of time we then spend wondering when people are going to start calling us "sir" or "miss," we fail to realize that this is as good as it gets internally. On average, after this time period is over, the slow decline begins. We begin to notice that it is hard to get as excited about life in general, that we aren't as full of energy as we used to be, and we wonder why that stupid alarm clock is ringing already. Didn't we just go to sleep?

One would hope it abates at a point, but, of course, it gets worse. The dreaded menopause and andropause (that's right, men; its coming for you, as well) hit us, and life in general can be pretty rough while we try to transition to having even less hormonal production. There is probably a joke in there somewhere about how **men**opause is the one that affects women, but we can thank the Greeks for ruining that (meaning cessation of month, in this case, monthly cycles).

As age keeps advancing, the systems in place for the creation of hormones are impacted throughout the body. Naturally, the levels cannot be maintained close to the ones of our youth. The means of production and conversion degrade over time along with the rest of our body. Hormones are not the sole part of us that is impacted either. Here is one example: The reason that many of us dislike the music kids listen to nowadays isn't simply because they have no taste in the really good stuff from back in the day but because of something that is at work in the body.

Dopamine is an important neurotransmitter (chemical created by nerve cells to send messages to other nerve cells) in our brain that is responsible for many things, one of them being our reaction to rewards or rewarding behavior. Studies show that when we listen to music that we like, even when we anticipate listening to music that we like, larger amounts of dopamine than normal are released in our brain.[2] Meanwhile, as the brain and body ages, the creation of dopamine significantly decreases.[3]

Now think back to the past when you were young. You were wearing your leg warmers or Members Only jacket, and you got so excited when the new Pat Benatar (or AC/DC, if you prefer) song came out. That flood of dopamine that you received when listening to your favorite music has slowly diminished over time because the overall level of it has diminished. Ultimately, you may like new music, but that "authentic" rush that you got when you were younger is lost to the ravages of time. This is partly the reason that "they don't make music like they used to." This also means that while we can keep yelling at teenagers about hormones, they can yell back at us for our "lame" dopamine.

It's not only about music. We simply brought it up because it is an easily associated change that happens with age. Perhaps they "don't make ice cream like they used to." Maybe you even miss the cafeteria food from school in the 1950s, despite the Hepatitis A you got from that place. Pleasurable experiences can decline with age due to the decreased amount of dopamine that you have in the old noggin. Going forward, keep this in mind and put it into context with any hormone that we will be looking at in depth. Maybe math is a little harder now; the old running legs aren't doing a lot of running nowadays. Yet, let's not get too far ahead of ourselves—time passes too quickly for us to waste time thinking about what we will talk about next when the present moment is devoted to discussing what exactly hormones are in the first place.

The Couriers of Life

Basically, a hormone is a chemical that acts as a messenger, manufactured by a cell to be transported to another cell. This prerequisite naturally excludes any single-celled organisms due to the nature of such an action, but all multi-cellular organisms contain hormones. Even the grass outside of your house is creating plant hormones when it isn't wondering when you will mow it again or when you will get rid of all those freeloading dandelions that moved in.

The actual word "hormone" derives from the Greek word for "impetus," which the dictionary defines as "driving force, impulse, or stimulus." This is quite the apt description for the ridiculous range of abilities and influences that hormones have. Small quantities of hormones can have a great effect on cellular metabolism, cracking the whip, so to speak, and getting everything in gear. After hormones reach a target cell, they bind to receptors either inside the cell or within the cell membrane, after which the cellular response is initiated.

The endocrine glands in the body have the main job of hormone production, and they release hormones directly into the bloodstream to their target destinations. Major endocrine glands are the pineal gland, the pituitary gland, the thyroid gland, the adrenal gland, the pancreas, and the gonads (ovaries in females and testes in males). The hormones created from these glands fuel the upcoming discussion, and they feature a prominent part in the restorative medicine approach.

Hormones themselves can be broken up into two different categories based on their chemical makeup. *Peptide hormones* are formed from chains of amino acids and include staples like insulin, growth hormones, and prolactin. *Lipid and phospholipid hormones* are derived from lipids and include steroid hormones, which themselves include the familiar heavyweights: testosterone and estrogens.

Although we are on the subject of chemical messengers, we will also include an observation of monoamines. These potent neurotransmitters include key players like melatonin, serotonin, and the previously mentioned dopamine. These chemicals should most certainly be considered when we look at a restorative approach to medicine. After all, it would be nice if we could come to appreciate that hullabaloo that our children call "sweet tunes" and if vanilla ice cream could once again taste like true vanilla ice cream by Jove! For now, we focus on the heavy artillery: the steroid hormones.

Simplified Chain of Steroid Hormone Production and Conversion

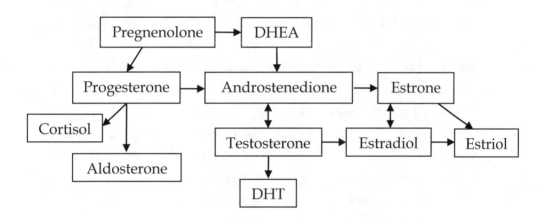

In this diagram, the arrows represent the route of conversion, in which one hormone turns into another. What is important to note about this flow chart, other than the fact it looks like a spider web constructed by an arachnid under the influence of caffeine, is that, much like the name implies, it is extremely simplified. For example, between pregnenolone and DHEA (*Dehydroepiandrosterone*, which is why nobody is willing to write out the name each time we mention it), there is an intermediate by the name of *17a-hydroxypregnenolone*. Another example is that progesterone does not convert directly into cortisol, but must first become *11-deoxycorticosterone*, then corticosterone, and then cortisol. We are also neglecting to mention the actual enzymes that carry out these conversion steps because we don't want to fill your head with names like *3β-hydroxysteroid dehydrogenase*. (Science, why are you so complicated? We love you, but you can be so difficult sometimes!) What we want to focus on are the actual steroid hormones.

We can group steroid hormones into five groups due to the receptors to which they bind. The groups are glucocorticoids, mineralocorticoids, androgens, estrogens, and progestogens. Glucocorticoids are present in almost all cells because they are responsible for important functions, such as immune response and metabolic activity. The beginning of the word refers to glucose because these hormones serve to keep blood glucose concentrations stable. Mineralocorticoids are hormones that have important functions in maintaining the balance between sodium, potassium, and water, which leads to them having an extremely important role in blood pressure regulation. Next, androgens are steroid hormones responsible for male characteristics. Likewise, estrogens are the primary hormones of the female sex. Progestogens include progesterone, which plays important roles in both pregnancy and the menstrual cycle, among many others, but is also present in men in smaller quantities.

That last bit might confuse some people. After all, many men are manly men and getting pregnant certainly isn't on the list of some burly lumberjack. He is concerned with chopping down the forest, not conceiving a child. Also, he has no uterus. This is where the label of "female" and "male" hormones sticks out like a sore thumb. Both sexes have the hormones; it is only a matter of differing qualities. Testosterone, the "manly" hormone that drives men to fell trees and burn up the dance floor in elaborate courtship rituals, is also present in women in much smaller quantities. However, as we will point out later, even though women might have a small level of testosterone overall, it does not mean that a decrease in this small level will not have sizeable impacts in certain areas.

Now that we have covered a bit of the background behind the hormones, we can look at the actual hormones that play a large role in our approach to restorative medicine. This is intended as a showcase for the power and potential of hormones. More digestible lists of symptoms and issues are available in the next chapter for easy reference.

Pregnenolone, the Grandfather of All

There goes that gender-based hormonal language again. We could have called pregnenolone the grandmother of all, but then we don't win with that either. Perhaps we can refer to pregnenolone as the grandparent of all. So, pregnenolone, the steroid hormone seen previously in the chart at the point of origin for conversion for the others, hence the moniker we have given it. Although pregnenolone is not a household name, it is nonetheless a very important hormone that seems to be ignored in public discourse relating to all things hormonal, which is a shame really, not to mention a horrifically grave oversight.

Pregnenolone is also the first hormone that we will be looking at that belongs not only to the steroid hormone family, but also to the neuroactive steroid classification. For simplicity's sake, these are often called *neurosteroids*. Neurosteroids are key players in the inner workings of the nervous system because they can influence the excitability of neurons.[4] On the whole, neurons tend to be quite an excitable bunch. When neurons communicate, they shoot out messages through chemicals and electricity. Unfortunately, this does not give us lightning-based magic or super powers, but it does mean that impulses and messages travel along your nervous system at breakneck speeds.

For example, move your arm up and down. You didn't just think, 'Okay, time to move my arm . . . Okay, I am starting to flex these muscles to raise my arm up and down, and, hooray, I am now moving my arm up and down.' Of course, that's not how it happened. You read the words, you moved your arm, and all is good in the world because you didn't have to think, you just did it. Now, our neurons do not simply exist for us to move our arm around while trying to figure out the inner workings of such an action. They are responsible for our daily functions that enable us to live. It's easy, then, to see how hormones, which are already entrenched on the cellular level like guerrillas in the mountain, that affect the nervous system are even more important than we give them credit for.

We can't neglect to reiterate that neurosteroids **control** excitability and do not simply **excite**. Our ability to respond to stimuli in a timely fashion and to react to impulses quickly is very important, but being able to tone down and "chill out" is just as important.

What about pregnenolone and the nerves? Are we just content to say that a neurosteroids are exceptionally good for having a well-oiled nervous system? Certainly not. There is, of course, more. We can look at specific instances where the presence or lack thereof of pregnenolone ties in with the functionality of a neurosteroid. We must never forget that although we can attribute the noun "nerves" to tangible and intangible concepts, the control center of the body is the brain, which is composed of a staggering amount of neurons (more than 80 billion of them).[5] Although impaired nerves in the body can lead to milder issues like the occasional twitch or a slowed reflex, impaired neural activity in the brain can lead to serious mental impairments.

Elderly patients with dementia have been observed to have low pregnenolone levels.[6] Many of us are familiar with the term "dementia", but in practical application, dementia is watered down in popular perception. Dementia is the decrease in mental function that is outside the realm of normal aging. Think of it as the difference between grandpa misplacing his book and then remembering that he left it out on the veranda. Hopefully, the situation isn't worse and doesn't entail grandpa permanently forgetting where he buried that chest of gold that was to be your inheritance (in which case we would also assume that your grandpa also forgot to tell you about his scurvy-fighting days as a pirate). Dementia does not necessarily have to manifest in severity; it can include some minor overall trouble with cognition. Unfortunately, dementia often originates from degenerative issues and gets worse as time goes on. Misplacing the keys can turn into misplacing your location in time and space. Alzheimer's disease is a familiar form of dementia.

Impaired mental function is not solely associated with progressive mental decline that results from aging. Generalized anxiety disorder is one such example, a condition categorized by excess mental worry greater than the actual source, which can manifest itself further in physical issues, including fatigue, nausea, and insomnia. Men with generalized anxiety disorder have been observed as having lower levels of pregnenolone than those in control groups.[7] This condition is the most common disorder in the workplace and is highly debilitating, with a high co-frequency of depression and other anxiety issues.[8] Margin trading stock brokers and employees of corporations who don't "believe in raises" can most probably relate.

A lack of pregnenolone has also been seen in individuals suffering from good old-fashioned depression as well.[9] Nobody really needs an introduction to depression since everyone has almost certainly been afflicted by it at some point or another. Although the natural reaction is to disagree, we have to remember that depression is the catchall label for all manner of depressive issues. It can be of the mild, transient variety like the time a crack commando squad of strawberry bud weevils infiltrated your potted garden on the terrace and destroyed your crop. On the other hand, it can be of the severe clinical depression variety, the one with serious issues, such as insomnia or suicidal thoughts after an ex-girlfriend burned the person's first edition printing of *Harry Potter*. What we can say as a blanket statement is that depression covers the wide range of depressed or low moods. At this point, pregnenolone has asked us to mention that it is also a player in mood control itself.[10]

Supplementation of pregnenolone has been shown to improve the body's response to stress.[11] Someone should probably tell that to those generalized anxiety guys. Pregnenolone also has indications for benefits in areas like arthritis, immune system function, and heart health. It is important to remember that we don't lightly crown pregnenolone with the title "grandparent." Conversion plays a large role in the creation of steroid hormone production. If there is not enough pregnenolone to go around for conversion into the next steps, then other areas will naturally suffer. To an extent, a deficiency in the previous tier of hormones can cause a deficiency in the current tier. If we're running a tin can-producing operation and start to run low on tin, then things are going to get hairy real fast.

DHEA, Ambiguously Manly

When we speak of DHEA, we usually go the quick and steady route of thinking that it's some kind of powerhouse that pushes us to great feats of strength and endurance. This wouldn't be too far from the mark. After all, we've heard all about how the testing committee in charge of ferreting out dopers and steroid users at the Olympic Games bans DHEA. So, how about the link between DHEA and all things physical?

First, we have to note that DHEA binds to androgen receptors, thus already giving it "street cred" in regards to its interaction with the physical realm. As we mentioned earlier, androgens are "male" hormones and have a close link with activity. In fact, exercising regularly has been shown to increase DHEA levels.[12] DHEA also happens to be the most proliferated steroid hormone in the body.[13] In regards to DHEA levels, one of two values is usually used: DHEA and DHEA-Sulfate (DHEA-S). DHEA-S is a metabolite of DHEA and can actually convert back into its precursor. Much more of DHEA-S can be found in the blood, which consequently provides a better gauge of how much DHEA is currently in the body. For this reason, the value of DHEA-S is often used for accurate readings.

DHEA is made primarily in the adrenal glands with other locations of production including the testes and brain.[14,15] One might point out to testes as being a male-only occurrence, and we would tend to agree. However, as far as androgens go, testosterone is the one that has a much greater ratio in men than in women, whereas in DHEA-Sulfate, the difference is certainly there, but not as pronounced. After all, women, being of the human species, have adrenal glands and brains just as men do (though some women might object about the latter for some specimens).

We prefer to shy away from going into deep detail about the glands responsible for hormone production because our focus is on the steroid hormones themselves. Therefore, let's look at the adrenal cortex for a specific example of interaction with DHEA. The adrenal gland is not limited to the production of just androgens, but also the glucocorticoids, mineralocorticoids, and corticosteroids. The gland comprises two parts: the cortex and medulla. The cortex can be seen as consisting of layers, in which the various hormones are produced. DHEA in particular is created in the innermost layer, the zona reticularis (you can purge this name from your memory, because there's no test at the end and it isn't a very interesting factoid to drop at your next cocktail party even if it is fun to say out loud). Now, decreased levels of DHEA in the body can lead to atrophy of this area.[16] "Atrophy" is one of those words that people don't wish to hear in conjunction with major organs.

As mentioned previously in regards to pregnenolone, there is the concept of decreased production throughout the tiers with steroid hormone interconversion. With DHEA in particular, we can easily see this in action. We already know that decreasing hormone levels because of a breakdown of functions is central to aging. Now, as DHEA levels decrease due to age, the production of androgens can decrease by half.[17] Let's shoot through the list of androgens again: DHEA, androstenedione, androstenediol, androsterone, testosterone, and dihydrotestosterone (DHT). If you look back at the chart in the beginning of the chapter, some of those are not present due to the simplification process. However, if you follow the full, non-simplified pathways down, all of the others originate from DHEA. If we observe a specific decade of life and compare it to what is optimal, for example, compare the 50-to-60-year-old range to the 20-to-30-year-old range, then we can see that DHEA levels decrease by 74 percent in men and by 70 percent in women.[18]

Another interesting action that just so happens to further discredit the concept of androgens as being male, is what happens to women post menopause. After the dreaded event occurs, almost all estrogens created in women are produced by conversion via DHEA. Even before menopause, this number can be as high as 70 percent. So, here we have DHEA, which is a "male" hormone, contributing in extremely large quantities to the most prominent "female" hormone. This is why gender labels for steroid hormones are bad, no matter how convenient they are, because they give people the wrong interpretation of hormones and contribute to preconceived notions about hormones seen as of the opposite gender. One would certainly not expect DHEA supplementation to aid older women in getting pregnant, but it does.[19] In fact, DHEA supplementation is used all around as an additional therapy when treating female infertility.[20]

We earlier covered how heart disease is a major killer, and DHEA is certainly no slouch in this department. Higher levels of DHEA-S have an association with better survival in cases of cardiovascular disease.[21] DHEA is classified as a neurosteroid, just like pregnenolone, and has a variety of associated benefits, particularly to improve levels. DHEA supplementation can cause improvements in memory, mood, and chronic depression.[22,23] When older individuals suffering from major depression and low DHEA-S levels were given DHEA supplementation to bring up their levels to more youthful ones, both their depression and memory improved in conjunction with the increased levels of DHEA-S and DHEA (don't forget that these can convert into each other). [24]

As fascinating as DHEA is, that's enough about this particular all-around powerhouse because we have more to cover. In the interest of knocking out androgens quickly so that we can move on to "female" hormones, we will be looking at testosterone next.

Testosterone, the Lumberjack Hormone

Testosterone, then, is the "mighty male hormone." It's testosterone that starts fisticuffs and fights in wars. It's testosterone that makes men build large objects that most certainly are not any form of compensation. It's testosterone that is produced in the ovaries. Wait, that last one seems a bit off. Of course, you are now well aware of our ploy to discredit gender labels on hormones. Obviously, testosterone is produced in the ovaries because women don't have testes (which are the main production area in men to the surprise of absolutely nobody).

After some snickering that is reminiscent of the sexual education classroom in middle school, a time period awkward for everybody, one naturally wants to tie in libido and sexual drive with testosterone. After all, with the testes, ovaries, and whatnot, it would make sense and would certainly be correct. The function of the aforementioned organs is to propagate the species. Accordingly, it is certainly natural that a hormone produced there would play a large part in the act.

Naturally, we wouldn't be likely to call testosterone the "lumberjack hormone" without putting in a comment somewhere about morning wood. There is a clear link between testosterone levels and male "potency", as well as a strong link between low levels of testosterone and erectile dysfunction. Men who received testosterone supplementation had improved sexual function.[25] Based on our previous mention that ovaries produce testosterone in women, it makes sense that testosterone supplementation helped women suffering from sexual dysfunction.[26]

We have been putting a lot of focus on dispelling the myth of male hormone specificity, but what gave androgens, and especially testosterone, such a male-focused leaning? A large part of it has to do with the final stages of male development before the full transition into adulthood. These final developmental stages include: the maturation of bone growth, increase in body and facial hair, and increased muscle mass and strength. In short, this is everything that begins to define the human male as a full adult man. This can certainly cross over into the female realm, as well.

The female breast, for example, is largely composed of adipose tissue, which in turn, is mostly fat (but not fully). Estrogens play a role in the development of breasts, which is largely negated in men due to their high testosterone levels (in part, due to the fact that testosterone helps prevent fat accumulation). However, in the example of female bodybuilders on the extreme end of the professional competition category, the breasts as visible anatomical entities begin to greatly decline while muscle mass increases in great proportion and overall body fat decreases. Granted, these are extreme cases that are frequently associated with pharmaceutical approaches to increasing testosterone levels, but it does show that to look like a typical man, one does not necessarily have to be a man. Even the anatomic feature colloquially known as "man jaw" can come about which is also aided by testosterone's role in decreasing fat layers deep beneath the skin in the human face.

Clearly, testosterone plays a large part in muscle growth and health. Now, there is also that important muscle in our chest beating an average of 70 times per minute. In one particular study, men who suffered from coronary artery disease had a correlation between low testosterone values and decreased survival.[27] Such studies on the nature of heart disease and testosterone mainly focus on men because even the scientific approach is not immune to gender labeling of hormones. In one study, made only of women with chronic heart failure, testosterone supplementation was seen as a potential treatment option.[28]

Does that wrap up the coverage of testosterone? Not quite. The more you know and all that, right? It seems that testosterone, when it isn't responsible for defending ancient Greece from a Persian invasion, has a knack for making the brain work well. Supplementation of testosterone has been shown to help improve neurons suffering from inadequate function. As a example of the correlation between testosterone and brain function, people who have Lou Gehrig's disease have been observed as having lower levels of testosterone.[29] Unfortunately, this disease (amyotrophic lateral sclerosis) does not turn a person into a baseball powerhouse, but instead causes deterioration of motor neurons (the neurons that control voluntary movement in the body), which is followed by death primarily from respiratory failure.

Estrogens, the Many as One

Those in the know might immediately recognize the plural of everyone's favorite female hormone, but others might be confused why it's "estrogens" and not "estrogen." Also, these people clearly skipped over the beginning of this chapter where there was no estrogen in the flow chart. Although there are many estrogens circulating out and about, the primary players are estrone (E1), estradiol (E2), and estriol (E3). In this instance, we use the term "key players" not to describe notoriety but through actual circulating amount—these three combined make up the bulk of estrogens in the body.

Because estrogens can be seen as the natural opposite of testosterone, their function in the development of the female body goes without saying. Estrogens are indeed responsible for the maturation of female secondary sex characteristics, such as breast development, the widening of hips, and the accumulation of fat in certain areas. Estrogens also play a large role in the function of the female reproductive system. You know it's coming . . . Again, we cannot fall into the gender hormone trap. Estrogen actually has an important role in male reproduction. Estradiol, in particular, helps prevent the apoptosis (programmed cell death) of sperm cells.[30] Remember, men, the next time you successfully help make a baby because not too many of your soldiers died off in the interim, you can thank estradiol.

Fluctuating levels of estrogens and progesterone help keep the monthly cycles regular. The concept of balance between estrogen and progesterone is something we will cover when we introduce the latter. During the regular 28-day monthly cycle of menstruation, estrogen goes up to peak levels towards the middle of the cycle in conjunction with ovulation (the process of egg release) and then drops off and hits the lowest amount prior to and during menstruation. The process repeats again until the cycle breaks with the onset of menopause.

The link between estrogen and bone health is perhaps a more subtle one. At the rate at which we see commercials on television about osteoporosis, focused entirely on women, we might as well have men high-fiving each other in the background while complimenting each other on their robust skeletal architecture. Osteoporosis hardly needs an introduction, being a well-known disease that decreases bone mineral density, making the bones more liable to break.

Another prominent fact is that the best state to have bones in is the unbroken state. Yet, we all know about great-grandma's walker with the tennis balls cut in half on the bottom, but we might not know particularly that bones are constantly broken down for parts (to put it crudely) and reformed. During osteoporosis, this normally healthy ratio of breakdown and creation is tilted toward the destructive process. Lower levels of estrogens load the dice in favor of the breakdown process.

Bones and reproduction aside, we cannot let the estrogens get away without mentioning the beneficial effect they can have on our old friends, the neurons. At this rate, you might think, 'Of course, they have an impact on neural activity, what steroid hormone doesn't?" We would tend to agree with that. Estrogen therapy during and after menopause seems to fare very well when braving the turbulent waters of impending Alzheimer's disease.[31] Restoration of estrogens to optimal levels helps women recover from depressions after child birth, during the process of menopause, and post menopause.[32] When women are afflicted with such types of depression, the public branding is to call them "hormonal." Whereas, a title that rings more true would be "big old lack of hormonal." Yes, men, women are often not hormonal enough.

Progesterone, the Great Stabilizer

Progesterone gets a bit of a diminished reputation, and unfairly so, because a large part of its efforts are aimed at helping balance out against estrogen. This is definitely true, as far as major functions of progesterone go. Yet, if we have learned anything so far, it is that no hormone operates solely based on the assumptions that people have about them. Although we are speaking of the mediating properties of progesterone, we should cover an important aspect in the restorative medical approach when it comes to these two "female" hormones.

Progesterone fluctuates based on the monthly cycle just as estrogen does. Unlike estrogen, progesterone gradually increases and then spikes in the later part of the cycle. However, it does drop off drastically like estrogen does just prior to menstruation. The regular cycle is part of the monthly balancing act, but a much larger balancing game is afoot in overall levels. Premenstrual syndrome, the scourge of women everywhere and better known as PMS, is related to the fluctuations of progesterone. This brings up the concept of estrogen dominance or progesterone dominance.

We must stress the dominance part of this terminology. The term "dominant" does not specifically mean "large" or "high" in the grand scheme of things. For example, let's say that in a local area, a group of cotton farmers all had their crop output horribly maimed by a plague-worthy infestation of boll weevils (weevils that eat cotton buds and flowers). One of these farmers turns out with the dominant amount of production in his cotton crop, but since everyone's output is greatly diminished, this "domination" works out in small numbers. In a better time, a good year with bumper crops, if that same farmer has the most production he will dominate again, but with high levels all around the board. Regardless of the overall levels, "dominant" simply means the highest in that group, regardless of the group size.

This is the exact same concept at work here, except we have progesterone and estrogens at work with each other. There's a whole different matter of ratios going on. There are issues associated with low progesterone and/or estrogens, as well as with high progesterone and/or estrogens. Still, then there are issues associated with dominance of progesterone or estrogens. So, let's say a woman has a low level of progesterone and a high level of estrogens. She would get issues associated with a low level of progesterone, potential issues associated with high levels of estrogens, and then, to sweeten the unsavory pot, issues associated with estrogen dominance (though, in this case, the issues of estrogen dominance would likely overshadow issues of high estrogens). Take the same woman and make the estrogens level lower than the progesterone, and she would have issues associated with low progesterone, low estrogen, and progesterone dominance. The level of progesterone in women tends to decline faster with age than that of estrogen, which means that this particular age-related decline favors the condition of estrogen dominance rather than progesterone dominance. Like all processes in the body with many variables, this is not always iron clad but is mostly the case. For ease of reference for these variables, we will knock out a proper list when we take a closer look at the restorative approach.

Neurons are never disappointed when progesterone is around because it can provide a benefit to mental function and can calm the nervous system. It has been observed that women who had Parkinson's disease had fluctuating symptoms based on what stage of their menstrual cycle they were in, and notable differences have been found in pregnant women.[33] Progesterone plays a very important role in allowing women to get pregnant and carry out to full term with very high increases in progesterone levels. Furthermore, progesterone supplementation can improve the outcome of brain and central nervous system injuries through limitation of damage, decrease of nerve tissue loss, and improved recovery time.[34] One might say that all of those are more than a bit beneficial when dealing with recovery from injuries of this sort.

We certainly could not let the last "female" hormone go without seeing how it specifically affects men, a tradition of sorts at this point. Much like estradiol, progesterone steps up to the plate by assisting in male reproductive efficacy. Although estradiol helps prevent the death of the "soldiers" marching on, progesterone plays a role in actually creating them.[35] Don't get us wrong, too many estrogens in the male body isn't a great thing and can lead to some negative effects, but all things in moderation, as they say. No man can say, "I'm a man, boy, and I ain't got none of them female hormones in my body," because yes, they do. If anything, a crude locker room jab at a man having trouble creating children can go something along the lines of "Hah, I bet that guy's progesterone and estrogen are in the dumps."

Cortisol, Stockbroker's Delight

The first impression that many people get when they hear the word "cortisol" is "that cream I put on my rash," but, of course, it wouldn't be mentioned in this section if it wasn't naturally produced in your body (also the common cream in reference here is referred to as hydrocortisone). Cortisol is frequently referred to as "the stress hormone" because levels are increased when the body is under stress, which also makes it the self-explanatory-labeled hormone. We would say we are happy to come up to another steroid hormone that is gender neutral, but now we have to deal with the "stress hormone" label. This is certainly an apt description of its well-known association, but sells short the variability of functions that cortisol is part of. The "establishment" just keeps on putting labels on everything.

Cortisol is produced in the cortex of the adrenal gland, in a layer more outward than the inner one that produces DHEA. Aside from stress response, it helps with the regulation of blood pressure and cardiovascular function, helps control metabolic activity and the breakdown of fats, carbohydrates, and proteins. Additionally, it helps suppress, the immune system. Yes, suppress. Now, such a function might seem to do more harm than good (or no good, for that matter), but we have to consider all the factors.

The human immune system is very loyal to us and efficient, but one might say it isn't too bright and can sometimes go off the deep end. Inflammation in the body is actually the response of the immune system trying to "right wrongs," as it were. However, sometimes the immune response is a bit too zealous in its approach to protecting the body, and the benefits of a moderating agent become readily apparent. Cortisol isn't trying to make you become sick easier; it's trying to reign in the overeager employees in the human body.

Cortisol, like progesterone and estrogen in women, is a fluctuating hormone (in both genders). Instead of a monthly cycle, it has a daily cycle with the highest amounts of it present in the morning. When we discuss symptoms of high or low cortisol levels, it is important to look at them in the context of long-term levels. One does not simply get the issues associated with low or high cortisol due to its daily fluctuations. When high and low cortisol levels are referred to, the reference is actually to a prolonged state of high or low cortisol levels in the blood. For example, hair loss is an issue of chronic high cortisol levels, not an issue of when cortisol is high in the morning. Thank goodness.

Now that we have covered the important steroid hormones, we can move on to our long-awaited and much anticipated restorative approach.

Optimized physiologic function is akin to Asclepius bringing in really good healing. Nine out of ten Greek doctors agree.

PART IV

On the Nature of the Restorative Approach

So, we spent some time going over some fundamentals about the body and medicine, but where does our particular approach of "restorative medicine" fit into this? We are glad you asked (after reading that question). The main concept to remember here is that while we showed some problematic areas with conventional medicine, by no means do we eschew conventional medicine. Despite any shortcomings, it is so widespread because it works in so many ways, as we explained earlier.

Secondly, this approach to restorative medicine only works because we co-operate with conventional, fully licensed and accredited doctors. There isn't a cadre of hedge wizards and nutritionists working on creating this approach based on the latest popular alternative health fad or on what "breakthrough" supplement the health magazines are trying to push. Instead, we take a rigorous, scientific approach toward observable variables, existing medical literature, and a comprehensive look at how the body works and how it fails. This approach is made solely while under the overseeing eyes of physicians of the licensed kind. So how does it begin?

Well, in accordance to scientific approach, there needs to be scientific assessment. We will go into depth about the restoration of the human body to optimal levels in order to help you have a full understanding, as well as the knowledge-derived ability to restore your good health. Once your understanding is achieved, individuals wishing to partake in our restorative approach must first fill out a detailed health history of past and current issues and symptoms. This inquiry is very detailed in the areas that we assess for our approach and is fully examined. Minute details that may not mean much to the layperson can divulge a lot of information to the trained eye. However, an approach focused solely on written accounts of symptoms and issues certainly tells us a lot, but it isn't exactly the best way to create a program. What's the best way to assess the condition of someone in a particular area? You got it. It's a test! In this case, a blood test.

The blood test is extremely important because while the knowledge is available to discern symptoms and descriptions of issues, actual data obtained from a blood test will help paint a much clearer picture of what is going on with regards to a suboptimal physiology.

The tests assess the following areas:

- ❖ **Lipid Profile**
- ❖ **Complete Blood Count (CBC)**
- ❖ **Comprehensive Metabolic Panel (CMP)**
- ❖ **Pregnenolone**
- ❖ **DHEA-Sulfate**
- ❖ **Total Testosterone**
- ❖ **Progesterone**
- ❖ **Total Estrogen**
- ❖ **Cortisol**
- ❖ **Thyroid Stimulating Hormone (TSH)**
- ❖ **Total Triiodothyronine (T3)**
- ❖ **Total Thyroxine (T4)**

- ❖ Prolactin
- ❖ Serotonin
- ❖ 25-Hydroxy Vitamin D
- ❖ C-Reactive Protein
- ❖ Homocysteine
- ❖ Prostate Specific Antigen (PSA)
- ❖ Insulin-like Growth Factor (IGF-1)
- ❖ Aldosterone

Using the data gleamed from these blood tests, a physician-approved program is created that consists of bio-identical hormones, supplements, and vitamins. This assembled product is individually created for each person because, believe it or not, each person's body is individualized. To find two individuals of the same age and gender having the exact same blood test results is an aberration of untold rarity and, from a practical and logical approach, will never be observed across the board. Granted, if someone orchestrates a plan so that all roughly seven billion humans on the planet can take a blood test and then puts that data into a computer network, we might find some. Until then, we'll just repeat the fact that, for optimal results, a blanket approach cannot be used.

People who are on medications may be required to stay on those medications, but over time, they may find that they do not need them anymore because of improved symptoms. With doctor approval and guidance, they can potentially discontinue them. This is especially true of cholesterol-lowering medications because this approach to restoration of function normalizes cholesterol levels naturally (we will get to that in a bit). Other examples include drugs for depression, insomnia, and erectile dysfunction (among many others).

Other than the individualized approach to program creation, the most important part of a successful program is constant feedback from the individual. People following our approach can login to an internet system (or call in Alexander Graham Bell fashion) to provide updates as frequently as needed to receive responses or program adjustments. This is in contrast to seeing a doctor and then seeing her again in a month or more, depending on how busy the office is. The consistent feedback and assessment allows for further customization and as-needed changes. The program is created in a tiered and modulated fashion so that any single item can be modified independently of others, which is partly the reason we stay away from multi-formula compounds like nobles from the peasant's quarter during a plague outbreak.

Another reason for our continual interaction with you is that on regular intervals, we ask for a follow up blood test to see what effect the program is having on the various levels (other than the effects that are already noted through frequent updates in the form of symptoms). Once these tests are received, the program may be modified. Even with a vast amount of experience in creating individualized programs based on the many factors obtained prior to creation, the rate at which an individual's body absorbs the agents or gets kick-started into creating its own is always variable because no two people have the same increases. The full explanation of the second reason is that if a multi-formula compound approach was used, this program adjustment and program adjustments in general would quickly become an exercise in futility.

Let's say that two systems are used, one with compounded agents and one with only single agents. The patient updates the doctor with an issue or a blood test result. In both cases, the doctor would say, this is the likely cause; let's modify this amount and see if the issue improves. The doctor using the single compound will be able to fix it up right as rain, but the doctor using a compounded agent will be up that certain proverbial creek with no paddle. A modification cannot be made without changing the entire compounded agent, which becomes an immense hassle and an extreme money waster. If there is one thing that's worse than a hassle, then that is a hassle that makes us spend more money.

To sum up: observations and descriptions of symptoms are assessed along with blood test results to create an individualized program under the guidance and control of a licensed physician that is then adjusted as needed based on feedback provided by the user and regular follow up blood testing. There are likely questions still on your mind: What are all those tests for? Isn't taking hormones dangerous? What exactly constitutes the items on the program? All these questions and more will be covered in the next sections. Should you want to peruse more information on the mystical engine dubbed by some the World Wide Web, you can find our website in the introduction. There is even a number to speak to an actual human and not a sinister "press 1 to continue" robot. Let's begin with some brief test explanations while also covering some of the symptoms associated with hormonal deficiencies.

The Vampire's Favorite Tests

Lipid Profile — Odds are that many people are familiar with this blood test since it comes standard on many blood requisition forms. This is simply a measure of total cholesterol, low-density lipoproteins (LDL), high-density lipoproteins (HDL), and triglycerides. Obviously, this is public enemy number one right now and is addressed by the restorative approach to medicine. We will go much further into detail about cholesterol in the next chapter.

Complete Blood Count (CBC) — This is the complete but also comprehensive blood test of your blood. That may sound awkward, but it is that self-explanatory. All the other tests are measuring specifically for certain particles floating about the blood, but this test measures the components of blood itself. We can roughly describe this as a measure of the red blood cells, the white blood cells, and the platelets and their subcategories. For example, in the realm of the red blood cells, the testing includes checking hemoglobin to assess the oxygen-carrying capacity of the blood and to check for conditions, such as anemia, as well as checking for things like the average width of red blood cells. As many learned in high school biology, white blood cells are the defenders of the body, and naturally their subcategories relate to such events if elevated. A simple example is eosinophil granulocytes, which can point to a possible parasitic infestation, asthma, or allergic reaction. Platelets are platelets, and this test can describe how "thin" the blood is, "thin" referring to the clotting capacity of the blood.

Comprehensive Metabolic Panel (CMP) — This test, along with the two above, probably rounds up the usual ones that are familiar to most people. Basically, it can be separated into categories. Glucose and calcium stand in their own group to have their levels measured. Electrolytes include mainstays like sodium and potassium, which are best served balanced. The other tests variably check on functionality of the kidneys and liver. The compounds in these groups naturally elevate when certain functions of the mentioned organs are impaired, and it can be simple to check for indicators that something is wrong in these areas.

Pregnenolone — We covered the grandparent of the other steroid hormones previously and would simply like to repeat that although pregnenolone is not well known, its functions and impact on other hormone levels cannot be underestimated.

- Precursor of many other hormones
- Fights the effects of fatigue and stress
- Relieves arthritis pain
- Improves heart health
- Boosts the immune system
- Protects against coronary artery disease
- Improves mood and memory
- Vital for full brain function
- Protection against degenerative brain diseases

DHEA-Sulfate — As you might recall, this is simply a metabolite of DHEA that can convert back into it but is the better indicator of DHEA values floating about in the blood.

- Improves heart health
- Slows the onset or progression of diabetes
- Has beneficial impact on arthritis
- Reverses declining cognitive function
- Low levels associated with increased risk of breast, ovarian, and other site cancer
- Optimal levels associated with maximum immunity and metabolic efficiency
- Around 50 percent of total androgens in men are converted from DHEA

- Contributes to 70 percent of estrogens pre-menopause and almost 100 percent post
- Levels decreased from peak levels by 95 percent in many people by age 75

Total Testosterone — This particular test is used because the free testosterone levels are not as reliable for interpretation (you could have a high level of free testosterone but a low level of overall testosterone). Below the following list of testosterone functions will be lists of the symptoms associated with low testosterone and low androgens in general.

- Boosts the male and female libido
- Promotes heart health
- Helps prevent osteoporosis (in larger part in men)
- Increases muscle strength
- Helps control blood sugar
- Helps with mental concentration and improves mood
- Protects the brain against Alzheimer's disease

Symptoms of Low Testosterone

- ❖ Prolonged fatigue
- ❖ Memory issues
- ❖ Decreased libido
- ❖ Vaginal dryness
- ❖ Muscle weakness
- ❖ Heart palpitations
- ❖ Bone loss
- ❖ Incontinence
- ❖ Fibromyalgia
- ❖ Irritability or moodiness
- ❖ Mental fuzz

❖ Depression
❖ Decreased motivation
❖ Diminished feeling of well-being
❖ Poor self-esteem
❖ Thinning skin
❖ General aches and pains
❖ Insomnia
❖ More aggressive prostate cancer
❖ Loss of scalp hair

Symptoms of Low Androgens

❖ Emotionality
❖ Extra sensitivity to emotional and physical stress
❖ Poor self-esteem
❖ Poor stamina
❖ Poor sex drive
❖ Cardiovascular disease
❖ Osteoporosis

Progesterone—A primary female hormone; also present in men to a much smaller degree. In the majority of menopausal women, these values are extremely low.

- Stimulates urine production
- Calms down the central nervous system
- A natural antidepressant and tranquilizer
- Improves female libido
- Protects against cancer
- Boosts thyroid action
- Helps use rather than store body fat
- Helps prevent osteoporosis

Symptoms of Low Progesterone

- ❖ Infertility
- ❖ Thyroid dysfunction
- ❖ Depression
- ❖ Fibrocystic breasts
- ❖ Weight gain
- ❖ Gallbladder disease
- ❖ Low blood sugar
- ❖ Panic attacks
- ❖ Water retention
- ❖ Irregular menstrual cycle
- ❖ Blood clots during menstruation
- ❖ Magnesium deficiency
- ❖ Vaginal dryness
- ❖ Breast tenderness
- ❖ Painful and swollen breasts
- ❖ Swollen extremities (prior to menses)
- ❖ Excessive menstruation
- ❖ Premenstrual syndrome
- ❖ Cysts and cancers of the breasts and ovaries
- ❖ Fibroids and uterine cancer

Symptoms of Progesterone Deficiency

- ❖ Irregular menses
- ❖ Heavy bleeding
- ❖ Cramping
- ❖ Swollen breasts
- ❖ Low libido
- ❖ Excess emotionality
- ❖ Excess sensitivity
- ❖ Depression and nervousness
- ❖ Anxiety and irritability

❖ Mood swings
❖ Weight gain
❖ Restless sleep
❖ Headaches
❖ Premenstrual migraine
❖ Premenstrual syndrome
❖ Acne
❖ Mental fuzz
❖ Joint pain

Symptoms of Progesterone Dominance and Excess

❖ Swelling of breasts
❖ Increased symptoms of estrogen deficiency
❖ Gastrointestinal bloating
❖ Candida exacerbation
❖ Drowsiness and excess sleep
❖ Mild depression

Total Estrogen—Having made it abundantly clear that there is no single estrogen, it would be prudent to test for the three main estrogens together.

▪ Determine the female appearance
▪ Allow ovulation to occur
▪ Important in lubrication of the mucous membrane (around the eyes, mouth, and vagina)
▪ Stimulates the central nervous system
▪ Improves the quality of skin, bones, and muscle
▪ Improves brain function
▪ Retains water and salt
▪ Relieves menopausal symptoms
▪ Increases female life expectancy

- Shields against coronary artery disease
- Helps prevent osteoporosis
- Protects against Alzheimer's disease

Symptoms of Low Estrogens

- ❖ Droopy, reduced, or overly small breasts
- ❖ Dry mucous membranes
- ❖ Short menses or long menstrual cycle
- ❖ Inadequate or lack of menses
- ❖ Headaches and migraines during menstruation
- ❖ Hair loss
- ❖ Fatigue
- ❖ Poor sex drive
- ❖ Cardiovascular disease
- ❖ Osteoporosis

Symptoms of Estrogens Deficiency

- ❖ Hot flashes
- ❖ Loss of libido
- ❖ Painful intercourse
- ❖ Vaginal dryness/atrophy
- ❖ Yeast infections
- ❖ Anxiety
- ❖ Depression
- ❖ Loss of memory
- ❖ Foggy thinking
- ❖ Dry skin
- ❖ Headaches and migraines
- ❖ Insomnia
- ❖ Heart palpitations
- ❖ Muscle and joint pain

❖ Bone loss
❖ Low mood and energy

Symptoms of Estrogens Dominance and Excess

❖ Menstrual cramps
❖ Heavy and irregular menses
❖ Breast swelling and tenderness
❖ Loss of sex drive
❖ Fluid retention
❖ Migraines
❖ Bloating
❖ Depression
❖ Mood swings
❖ Nervousness, anxiety, and irritability
❖ Weight gain
❖ Fatigue
❖ Craving for sweets
❖ Hair loss
❖ Symptoms of low thyroid hormone
❖ Mental fuzz
❖ Fibrocystic breasts
❖ Uterine fibroids
❖ Endometriosis
❖ Hormone dependent cancers

As a clarification, we should mention that the difference between low and deficiency is a matter associated with age. Deficiency is the description of levels in old age when there is a chronic deficiency of hormones.

Cortisol – The "stress hormone."

Symptoms of High Cortisol

❖ Impaired mental performance
❖ Suppressed thyroid function
❖ Imbalances of glucose
❖ Decreased bone density and muscle tissue
❖ Increased blood pressure and abdominal fat
❖ Depression
❖ Sleep disturbances
❖ Low libido
❖ Anxiety
❖ Hair loss
❖ Elevated triglycerides

Symptoms of Low Cortisol

❖ Antisocial and criminal behavior
❖ Insomnia via adrenaline overload
❖ Heart palpitations
❖ Acne
❖ Fatigue
❖ Depression and panic attacks
❖ Irritability
❖ Infertility (via low progesterone)
❖ Migraines and headaches
❖ Fibromyalgia
❖ Cravings for sweets
❖ Allergies
❖ Chemical sensitivities
❖ Symptoms of low progesterone
❖ Symptoms of low thyroid hormone

TSH (Thyroid Stimulating Hormone) — Upon first glance, one might assume that this is a thyroid hormone but not quite. Note that it is the hormone that stimulates the thyroid, and it is produced by the pituitary gland. Basically, this hormone tells the thyroid to create thyroid hormones when levels of said hormones are low. If the levels are high, production of TSH decreases. In short, the production of TSH helps keep the thyroid hormones in balance. For the purpose of restorative medicine, optimized thyroid function is important because it regulates how sensitive the body is to hormones in general.

Total Triiodothyronine (T3) — The more active thyroid hormone. Has extremely important functions, such as the regulation of growth and development and heart rate, as well as assistance in metabolic and body temperature control. It has an effect on almost every physiological process in the body.

Total Thyroxine (T4) — Also plays a very important role in the body's metabolism, stimulating the consumption of oxygen in the body. T4 also converts into T3.

Thyroid Hormones

- Control cell growth and metabolism
- Help with weight management
- Improve heart and vascular health
- Renew energy
- Aid concentration
- Regulate body temperature

Symptoms of Low Thyroid Function

- ❖ Fatigue
- ❖ Cold extremities
- ❖ Low libido
- ❖ Dry skin
- ❖ General aches and pains
- ❖ Depression
- ❖ Scalp hair loss
- ❖ Brittle nails
- ❖ Low pulse and blood pressure
- ❖ Memory lapses
- ❖ Heart palpitations
- ❖ Constipation
- ❖ Low stamina
- ❖ Low body temperature
- ❖ Headaches
- ❖ Intolerance to cold
- ❖ Weight gain
- ❖ Anxiety
- ❖ Swollen, puffy eyes
- ❖ Poor concentration
- ❖ High cholesterol
- ❖ Infertility
- ❖ Fibromyalgia

C-Reactive Protein—Quite simply, this is a protein whose level increases when there is inflammation in the body. As such, it can be an indicator for a variety of ailments ranging from arthritis and cancer to heart disease.

Prolactin — Perhaps the most known function of prolactin is in the link it has to lactation. Increasing levels of prolactin stimulate lactation post pregnancy once progesterone levels have decreased. Outside of such scenarios, high levels of prolactin can point to issues like sexual disorders or lack of menstruation.

Serotonin — This is a very important neurotransmitter associated with feelings of well-being and happiness, as well as a host of other functions. Many classes of drugs, such as antidepressants and antipsychotics, alter serotonin levels. This also the case with many popular drugs used to treat anxiety.

25-Hydroxy Vitamin D — Although vitamin D is not technically a vitamin, it is nonetheless important in the human body. Mammals (and thus humans) synthesize vitamin D when sunlight hits the skin and can acquire it through dietary means. It can also have an influence on cholesterol production.

Prostate Specific Antigen (PSA) — This male-only test is for the measurement of PSA in the blood, elevated levels of which can potentially point to prostate cancer or an enlarged prostate.

Insulin-like Growth Factor (IGF-1) — This important protein has many functions, among them the regulation of the growth of nearly every cell in the body. Low levels of this protein can point to issues as serious as cardiovascular disease.

Homocysteine — This is an amino acid, high levels of which can point to an increased risk of cardiovascular disease.

Aldosterone — This test is not always performed, but the function of aldosterone cannot be denied. It is actually the most potent hormone in the body in regards to the balance of electrolytes. It has regulatory effects on the metabolism of carbohydrates, regulates blood pressure, and can be employed against low blood pressure, hearing loss, tinnitus, and migraines.

Factory Grade Hormones and Horse Urine

With the blood tests now covered, you might go the second question posed regarding the safety of taking hormones. The ones in your body are certainly on the straight and narrow, but what about the ones you actually take in? Certainly, many people have been showered with stories about hormones, their side effects, and other just all around bad things about hormones.

Well, perspective is always best gained from several directions. Let's first look at steroid hormones, which are produced in your body. Your body manufactures them, it uses them, and they are meant to be part of the overall human anatomical "ecosystem." However, that's definitely not the first association that pops into the minds of most people. The first thought is usually of "those other" steroids. Well, actually, there is no "those other steroids." It's just those synthetic anabolic steroids.

Synthetic anabolic steroids are drugs, key word being, of course, drugs, that are meant to imitate the effects of testosterone and dihydrotestosterone. Let's consider a former United States president and a person who looks a lot like this president and can talk like him. One of these individuals will provide a budget surplus while the other one is going to look and sound a lot like the president. Which one would you prefer running your country?

This is the problem with synthetic anabolic steroids and any drugs that try to mimic what we have in our bodies.

These synthetic substances do not have the same chemical formulas as the ones inside of our bodies because you can't patent the formula of the things in your body because that wouldn't make sense, and you couldn't charge the proverbial arm and leg for it either. One could, of course, always think, 'What's the problem with maybe a little extra carbon here, maybe a bit of oxygen over there in the chemical formula?' The thing is that your body creates the chemical formulas it does for a reason; they work and are specifically made to carry out their proper functions. Synthetic imitators are recognized as the dirty infiltrators that they are. The body does not fully accept them as a true replacement. Nothing is ever as good as the real thing.

Let's use a commonly known example: progestin, a synthetic progesterone often used various birth control pills. In one study, women who used estrogen and progestin had a significantly higher risk of acquiring breast cancer, but women who used progesterone that was bio-identical, or identical to the one found in the body, had a decreased risk of breast cancer.[1] Another study that tried a combination of non-bio-identical estrogens and progestin had to be stopped before running its course because risks for both heart attacks and breast cancer increased.[2]

There is another distinction that has to be made in regards to our usage of the term "bio-identical hormone." When we refer to the use of bio-identical hormone supplementation, we are referring to bio-identical for the *human* body. Premarin, a popular estrogen replacement that has fallen out of use lately because of published studies regarding risks like endometrial cancer,[3] is what you could technically call bio-identical. However, it is bio-identical in the sense that it comes from horses. To be more exact, estrogens derived from the urine of pregnant horses with part horse estrogen. Hence, the name - **PRE**gnant **MAR**es' ur**IN**e (someone get in touch with Interpol; we cracked the code). Now,

we can't go around claiming to be all knowing experts about everything, but "word on the street" is that the human body is not exactly lacking in its production capacity of estrogen derived from the urine of horses who maybe had too much to drink one night and didn't use protection.

And that's the problem. Popular perception and mental imprinting associates the words "steroids" and "hormones" not with the natural ones made in the body but with those synthetic ones, which from a chemical and biological standpoint do not belong in the body at all. When our ears hear "estrogen," our brains pull up all the bad things associated with pregnant mare urine extract (doesn't quite have the same ring as vanilla extract) and not the estrogens in our body. Reports and articles certainly don't help either with their liberal use of "estrogen" (and not even "estrogens") when the subject matter is about synthetic and not bio-identical hormones. But, hey, who needs journalistic integrity and editorial fact checking when buzzwords and sensationalism sell articles?

Sealing the Compartments of a Sinking Ship

So, it is now understood that the individualized restoration approach covers both the hormones and the tests and creates a program for all the factors. How does the spread go? The most important thing to remember is the one-to-one approach. Pregnenolone for pregnenolone, DHEA for DHEA, and so on and so forth, and not mixtures, such as, say, combined pregnenolone and DHEA. Everything from the hormonal side is approached via the oral route excepting progesterone, estrogens, and the testosterone.

Now, ordinarily, the oral route is seen as a rather inflexible approach, and we would agree in the case of the last three hormones we just mentioned. However, in the case of something like pregnenolone, an oral route can easily be made modifiable. For example, let's say that based on the history and blood test, it is suggested that 75 milligrams of pregnenolone be used. The suggestion for a bottle of just 75 milligrams of pregnenolone would not be given. Instead, the power of mathematics is used in the consultation, and something like bottles of 50 milligrams and 25 milligrams would be suggested so that they can be taken together and easily increased or decreased as needed. This ability to modify is the approach taken with hormones of the oral sort.

The progesterone, estrogens, and testosterone approach is different. An oral route is not followed because it is too inflexible for these. The gel-in-syringes approach is much more conducive to our set intentions. Just to be perfectly clear, that is the syringe with gel that is squeezed out and rubbed onto the skin, not a syringe with a needle that injects gel into the body because that would be the definition of a bad time. This approach allows for the quick modulation of these hormones and better mirroring of the body's fluidity.

Part of the optimal female physiology during the early age is the cyclic nature of the menstrual period, which, as we mentioned, is caused by the fluctuation of progesterone and estrogens. The restorative approach takes this well into account and follows variable doses for the pattern of the menstrual cycle or via an artificial cycle for women post menopause. On top of the 1:1 hormone approach, there are other common components of the program.

Melatonin, Morpheus' Confederate

Melatonin is a hormone, a neurohormone and not a steroid hormone, hence its omission from the main bunch before. Melatonin is best known for is its function within the circadian rhythm. The circadian rhythm is certainly not a human-only phenomenon and can be found in animals, plants, and even bacteria. Basically, this rhythm is the description of biological function that differentiates depending on the time of the standard 24-hour day due to reactions from factors, such as daylight, in your environment.

Melatonin is also known as a "night" or "darkness"" hormone because it is created when such conditions occur. The pineal gland is its site of in the human body. It is an endocrine hormone and enters directly into the blood stream. When light enters the human eye, production of melatonin is suppressed. Don't mistakenly refer to melatonin as the "go to sleep" hormone because if there's one thing we've learned so far it is that hormonal labels are bad. Every single hormone seems to be an over-achiever and wants to do many different jobs. Melatonin is also a potent antioxidant (we will cover these beneficial agents at a later point) and plays a role in the cell death of cancers.[4] Furthermore, it is particularly good at its well-known job as a weapon in the battle against insomnia.

Magnesium, Brunch of Cellular Champions

Many people subconsciously accept the fact that the human body has some elements that do not seem like they belong there, such as iron in hemoglobin. Accordingly, there is not much recognition of the importance of metals and their functions in allowing us to live. Without the mentioned iron in our bloodstream, our body would not receive oxygen, and oxygen is most definitely something that Earth-dwelling organisms like to use. We accept that iron supplements help with iron-deficient anemia, but all the links on the cellular biological side are typically not fully considered. Such is the case with magnesium.

When most people think of magnesium as it applies to the human body, they are likely to think of milk of magnesia, the common name of magnesium hydroxide. Magnesium hydroxide has two general uses: as an antacid and as a laxative, the latter being the more well-known use. Suffice it to say, if a person is feeling "stopped up," a swig of the old milk of magnesia is likely to clear up even the most egregious of obstructions. Is that it? Is the sole role of magnesium to be a savior after a particularly over-indulgent night at an all-you-can-eat Brazilian steakhouse?

Enter adenosine triphosphate (ATP). We won't linger on ATP too long because the most important thing to know is that we can think of it as the energy unit of cellular metabolism. It is often called the energy currency of life because every cell has it and needs it. Mini high school biology refresher aside, what does this have to with magnesium? In order for mitochondria, the energy-producing organelles within cells, to function and produce more ATP, it first needs to be powered by magnesium-bound ATP.

How about that, magnesium? You just shot up from constipation aide to being absolutely vital for human survival.

Knowing this vital function of magnesium leads to no surprise at the variability and potential severity of symptoms resulting from improper levels: starting on the mild level with muscle cramps and fatigue, moving up to full on muscle spasms and nausea, all the way up to heart failure.[5-7]

Magnesium can have a calming effect on the nervous system and, as such, can be a great aid in helping with issues like headaches, migraines, and muscle spasms—and, yes, constipation, but magnesium doesn't appreciate being known only for that. Based on the symptoms and issues often presented in individuals who want to take the restorative medicine approach, the recommendation of magnesium is often a given. According to the Agricultural Research Service, which is part of the United States Department of Agriculture (USDA), 43 percent of the population in the United States receives adequate magnesium through diet, meaning of course that more than half do not.[8] We can safely say that the level of magnesium consumption in the United States is not "USDA choice."

Serotonin, Herald of Happiness

We already mentioned some of the benefits of serotonin, but wanted to stress that a different route must be taken in regards to oral administration. Essentially, the "blood brain barrier" is the term for the separation of the blood circulating in our bodies from the fluid surrounding our brain, which makes it so that everything does not go all over the place willy-nilly. This is a safeguard against foreign invaders, such as bacteria, but also grants entry to certain friends such as oxygen molecules and hormones.

Orally taken serotonin is not able to cross this barrier. Seeing as how the effects of serotonin as a neurotransmitter can certainly be useful in a brain composed entirely of neurons, this would be a problem. However, 5-Hydroxytryptophan (5-HTP) is a precursor of serotonin and melatonin that can in fact cross this blood brain barrier. An individual with an inadequacy of serotonin would not get a "serotonin" supplement" but rather 5-HTP instead. You can eat avocados all day long with their high serotonin content, but if it isn't getting through to the brain, then all that guacamole was eaten for naught; although the tortilla chip manufacturing industry does thank you. The majority of serotonin is actually found in your intestines, but its effects on the brain cannot be understated. Although serotonin binds to neurons and neurons can obviously be found throughout the body, the brain is a particularly important concentration of said neurons with many specific functions other than "Ouch! Fire hot!"

Intestinal Flora, the Great Absorbers

This term is code for the restoration of the good bacteria that live in your intestines at this very moment because they're in there, moving around, and helping you stay healthy (we apologize for the mental image of trillions of living organisms moving around in your bowels). Of course, the term "bacteria" usually brings to mind those disease-causing blighters, but there are a lot of good bacteria, especially in our gastrointestinal system. This restoration or optimization is accomplished by the taking of what is called "probiotics," a term certainly familiar to many people via yogurt commercials because if those commercials are to be believed, then when commercial actors aren't acting, they're chronically constipated and need probiotics to stay regular.

The well-known role of intestinal flora is in digestion and absorption. Although the stomach and intestines already do a bang up job in this department, the bacteria living in those parts help speed things along or even help us break down what we normally couldn't. A good example of this is termites. They don't just eat wood and digest it themselves; the relationship they have with the organisms in their gut allows them to digest the cellulose from the wood. In fact, the protozoa living there help with this function, and those protozoa themselves have symbiotic bacteria that help them in their function. It seems that termites have many more beneficial symbiotic associations than we give them credit for, which is hard to want to do when those little devils are eating one's brand new timber cottage. The bacteria in our human digestive system go after some carbohydrates, such as certain starches and fibers, because we lack certain enzymes for their digestion. Ultimately, through their actions, bacteria provide the human body with energy and nutrients that we would otherwise miss out on.

In addition to good digestion and absorption, intestinal flora is responsible for boosting our overall immune system by helping prevent the growth of pathogenic bacteria, the kind we certainly don't want in our digestive tract. This hefty "us or them" approach allows beneficial bacteria to flourish and bring in more of their type while trying to keep the bad ones out in the rain. Intestinal flora can also potentially help with allergy prevention and inflammatory bowel disease like with Crohn's disease. Serotonin is also produced in the intestines.

Keep in mind that when bad bacteria set up shop in our body, we are often prescribed antibiotics. Unfortunately, while the bacteria in our intestines have friend or foe targeting, the antibiotic won't be as discretionary. When the antibiotic goes to work, it gets down to business and likes to annihilate everything in its path. Yes, that tends to kill our foreign invaders, but not without casualties, for it does some serious Dresden bombing action on our civilian bacteria population. Hence, the reason antibiotics commonly cause diarrhea as a side effect is that your native Home Team population is suddenly at a disadvantage.

Saw Palmetto, Blocker of Receding Hairlines

When we say saw palmetto, we aren't referring to the leaves or some kind of ground up paste from saw palmetto, which is a type of palm. We specifically refer to the extract from the fruit of the saw palmetto. The reason for this is because it inhibits the actions of 5-alpha reductase. We generally try to stay away from enzyme names because the learned men behind their naming tried their utmost to keep them out of ordinary conversation with all their hyphens and most unnatural compositions.

So, back to the matter at hand, 5-alpha reductase is the enzyme that you would have seen in our chart as being the intermediary between testosterone and dihydrotestosterone (DHT). Why in the world would we want to tell 5-alpha to hold its reins here and there? To answer that question, we have to look at DHT.

DHT is extremely potent. If testosterone is the most cut and muscular guy at the gym benching 150 kilograms, then DHT is the bigger guy having a bit of a laugh as he prepares to do his set of 400 kilograms with no spotter (because he doesn't need one and will get angry if you suggest otherwise). Basically, anywhere testosterone can perform, DHT can outperform. It is more prone to attachment to testosterone receptors and is more potent overall, with about five percent of testosterone going over to become DHT. One might think, 'What's the big deal? If there is this super testosterone floating about, why would we not like that?'

Being bald comes to mind since DHT is the main culprit behind male pattern baldness, and, to a lesser extent, the female variety (more factors go into female hair loss). It is also a contributor to benign prostate hyperplasia (BPH) due to its effect on prostate enlargement.[9] BPH is simply code for the enlargement of the prostate gland without that nasty association of prostate cancer. Although there are certain parts of the groin region that some men would wish to enlarge, having a prostate swelling to grapefruit proportions is not what they have in mind.

DHT laughs at men in more ways. Consider the big picture, as we are always trying to do when speaking about how complex our body system is. You saw the side effects that can come with the age-related decline of hormone production, and now let's put some factors together. A man in the prime of his life starts to age in the bad direction because Mother Nature is out to get him. All those hormones begin to decline, and then the body thinks, 'Oh man, you have to listen to this because I have a great idea. Testosterone is falling, but we got that old boy DHT to save the day. He's way more potent than testosterone, which we don't have enough of anymore to be all man.'

Logically, the body then implements its great idea to produce more DHT through conversion. On paper, it makes sense because DHT is stronger and thus should technically pick up the slack by the lowered testosterone level. However, taking into consideration all the factors at play here including slowly elevating levels of estrogens in men as they age, this is not the best of ideas the body has had. In short, the "correction" of applying more potency backfires. What we wind up is not a favored bald movie star, as the body would believe it is making. No, what we wind up with is Uncle Mark in his grape-jelly-stained tank top, sweat pants, and sandals, who is afflicted by male pattern baldness, a pot belly, love handles gymnasts could hang on to for complex maneuvers, and a prostate that sends him to the urinal every ten minutes during your annual trip to Disney World.

Zinc, Catalyst and Man Keeper

Zinc plays many important roles in the body. These various performances include ensuring prostate gland function[10] and functioning as a widespread catalyst for many enzyme reactions, even in the metabolism of RNA and DNA, the keepers of our genetic information. It has even been shown to be part of an efficient treatment approach in age-related macular degeneration. We will cover macular degeneration in slightly more detail, but for now, it is a condition in which retinal damage slowly causes the afflicted to lose full use of their sight, sometimes even resulting in blindness.[11] Suffice it to say, the importance of zinc in processes of biological nature cannot be overstated.

For our purposes here, we would emphasize that zinc is employed in the hormonal restorative approach. If you go back up to the chart, you can put in the enzyme, aromatase, which converts testosterone into estrogens, between testosterone and estradiol. As men age, this process tends to increase. Although we made it clear that estrogens play important roles in men, men having too many estrogens are not good for them because such is the domain of women and symptoms of excess estrogens can hit men just as hard (say hello to your new friends, the love handles). Zinc factors into this because it works as an aromatase inhibitor.

Its application in the approach spreads across several levels. Older men who are having issues with elevated estrogens due to an excess of this conversion can benefit via lower levels of estrogens. Even obesity can make the process of aromatization kick into higher gear. Individuals using testosterone supplementation can benefit since it can prevent extra conversion from occurring.

As We Stand Here Amongst All These Old Trees

When you read all the information presented so far, you might have thought, 'But, no . . . My hormones are fine. I had a blood test recently and I actually checked some of these things out, and it said that I was fine and within my range for everything.' We will look at this next in order to fully clarify these ranges.

Take note that when reference ranges are mentioned, statistics rears its giant ugly head and starts grouping people. This is very nice because we need to have distinctions and subsets of populations so that we can accurately study all that is going on. However, in this case, this doesn't help us that much when we consider where we want to be at as opposed to where we are now.

Let's say that you are in your seventies and aren't as spry as a young elm tree anymore, and your daughter and her family are over to visit. This includes your favorite grandchildren, but, mercy me, those grandchildren just won't shut up and stop

running around. They keep asking you to play tag with them, but the jig is up because they have the advantage. Maybe your daughter told them about the will and testament that leaves them with the catfish farm and they want to expedite that process by giving you a heart attack. How else are they going to pay for college to get a degree that won't get them a job due to an unemployable major?

You feel old. You have plenty of friends your age at your local backgammon club, and they all feel old too. Some of them whisper fearfully that their grandchildren are out to get them, as well. You are seemingly past your prime, and you don't feel too hot because of that. However, you can see it now in your head, as clear as a dehydrated alcoholic stranded in the

Sahara sees a rum factory glimmering above the dunes, that all those test results are in "your range," but who is in your range?

Everyone at your backgammon club. Everyone who "feels their age" and feels just as old and worn out as you. This is your reference range. Now, look back to your twenties when you felt great, when birds were singing in the air, and the threat of communism loomed like a rapidly deflating hot air balloon. If you had checked your blood tests at that time (and were also a time traveler because some such tests did not exist back then), then you would have likely been in your reference range, as well.

At both times you would be in your reference range. The main difference is that at one end of that time, you are in the reference range during the prime of your life while on the other end, you are the reference range of "maybe I should go visit Paris because I can't remember where I buried my chest of gold anymore and that dumb farmer in a black robe keeps following me around and waving at me." Now, consider how you would like to feel—old and worn out or young and vigorous. To achieve some manner of restoration towards that energy and function, you would have to place yourself in the reference range of yourself as you were in your twenties and away from your backgammon club range.

This is the way that the restorative approach seeks to further its goals. What is the point of being at a good level according to your reference range when that range is meant to confine you to the level in which so much of your good functions from the Jazz Age are impaired? The approach seeks to restore your levels to those of a healthy person of your gender who is 20 to 29 years old. As we mentioned earlier, this is that golden time period when you can go trapping beavers on the frontier because you feel great, that time before all those pesky associations with low hormone levels begin to crop up due to your advancing age. What follows is the range then, the optimal one, and not the backgammon one.

Steroid Hormone Range for Women	Reference Range (20-29-year-old bracket)	The Optimal Range
Pregnenolone	10-230 ng/dL	157-230 ng/dL
Total Estrogen	61-437 pg/mL	150-437 pg/mL*
Progesterone	0.2-28 ng/mL	1-28 ng/mL*
DHEA-Sulfate	65-380 ug/dL	275-380 ug/dL
Total Testosterone	14-76 ng/dL	55-76 ng/dL
Cortisol (tested in the AM)	4.3-22.4 ug/dL	16.4-22.4 ug/dL

depends on the phase of the menstrual cycle

ng=nanograms pg=picogram ug=microgram dL=deciliter mL=milliliter

Steroid Hormone Range for Men	Reference Range (20-29-year-old bracket)	The Optimal Range
Pregnenolone	10-200 ng/dL	137-200 ng/dL
Total Testosterone	241-827 ng/dL	632-827 ng/dL
DHEA-Sulfate	280-640 ug/dL	520-640 ug/dL
Total Estrogen	0-130 pg/mL	<43 pg/mL
Progesterone	0.3-1.2 ng/mL	0.9-1.2 ng/mL
Cortisol (tested in the AM)	4.3-22.4 ug/dL	16.4-22.4 ug/dL

ng=nanograms pg=picogram ug=microgram dL=deciliter mL=milliliter

As seen in these charts, we have the reference range of the decade of life that we want to try and rekindle, as well as the optimal range. It stands to reason, based on issues associated with lower levels and benefits associated with higher levels, that simply being in the reference range is not fully indicative of the greatest benefit that can be received. After all, a pregnenolone level of 15 is within the reference range, but isn't exactly what one would want when trying to fight off possibly encroaching dementia. The only thing worse than having spiders in your room at night is forgetting whether you have spiders in your room at night. The optimal range is roughly the upper one-third of this reference range.

So, let's sum up how this all works:

- ❖ History of symptoms and issues is provided and assessed, blood tests are reviewed.
- ❖ A program to cover the issues is created while following several core tenants: convenience in regards to taking only what is needed the most, affordability, specific application against issues and values, wholly individualized for each person, and extreme modularity in program design for quick modification potential.
- ❖ The assessment of feedback from the user delivered frequently for possible program modification.
- ❖ Regular blood tests at varying intervals (three to six months) for further adjustments and assessment.

This is the summarized approach. In an earlier part, we already mentioned the issues associated with low levels of various hormones. We have also described symptoms of deficiency, imbalance, or excess when it comes to steroid hormones. We will also go into various other deficiencies and diseases that have an application in the restorative medicine approach.

At this point, you might be wondering about something important. We spoke at length about certain issues, but you may have noticed that something was lacking from the discussion, something that is on the mind of millions concerned with their health. Cholesterol was referenced earlier, but it seems like mum's the word now with nary a mention. This is because cholesterol is one to watch, a very important topic to discuss and we thought it important to devote some time to it. So let's take a look and see what cholesterol's deal is and why it seems to act like such a big jerk.

Cholesterol and Prometheus have some things in common. They achieved bad boy status while doing something good and then were hung in the court of public opinion.

PART V

On the Nature of Cholesterol

High cholesterol—the very phrase probably sends shivers up the spines of many, bringing about thoughts of something bad in our body slowly digging our grave at the local cemetery. Everywhere we turn, the eternal war against cholesterol rages on (and by eternal we mean starting late in the 20th century). A brief stroll through the grocery store shows those convenient butter-like substances that have low cholesterol, as well as certain breakfast cereals that have cholesterol-lowering properties. The friendly doctors and patients on all those television commercials seek to educate us by repeating that high cholesterol just might be responsible for buying us a first class ticket across the Styx. Why, even those nice people at the pharmaceutical companies are helping us out with lower prices on generic cholesterol-lowering drugs because their patent expired.

Well, it is very reassuring to all of us that so many people and companies care about our high cholesterol! However, some, or even many of us, may have questions. Rampant consumerism is certainly a wonderful teacher because if so many people spend so much money creating and advertising a way down from the Cholesterol Mountains, why then it must be a good idea. However, regardless of popular opinion, some people might want to throw caution into the wind and learn something for themselves. So, what about this cholesterol?

Well, we are so glad that inquiring minds want to know. Let's approach it from the most popular direction. We consume cholesterol in our daily food, the overindulgence of which can lead to greatly increased levels. Cholesterol levels are usually mentioned in tandem with triglycerides, after all, and triglycerides compromise a large part of fat in humans. Not to mention that all those cholesterol-lowering commercials are always talking about "along with diet and exercise." Cholesterol can indeed be what is termed "dietary cholesterol" or, simply put, cholesterol that we gain from food. However, dietary cholesterol makes up a small amount of our cholesterol. So where, then does the impish spawn come from?

Turns out that it is from our own bodies. Great, so not only is Mother Nature out to get us in general with that whole age thing while cars and television sets can increase our risk of heart disease, but now our own body is in on the whole scheme, as well. Okay, maybe that's a bit harsh. Perhaps the body is having a bad time or is under duress when it creates what seems like such a dangerous compound. Let's take a look at where this vile substance is in our bodies.

Let's start with the liver. Why the liver? Well, the liver is actually a production site of both triglycerides and cholesterol. Well that's nice; not only is the liver always on our case about keeping it healthy and begging us not to overindulge in the fruity alcoholic drinks, but now it has the audacity to manufacture that garbage in our bodies? The betrayal doesn't end there. The liver twists the proverbial dagger in our backs by not only creating cholesterol but also sending it out all throughout our bodies. It even takes some of it back in, reabsorbing it to create more of the vile stuff. Whatever, liver. You think you got the upper hand now, but we're taking this information to the head honcho. That's right, the jig is up because we are going to tell the brain all about your little plan here to kill off the body.

Hold on now; something seems off. The brain is tainted with cholesterol, as well. Heavens to Betsy, what in the name of Nikola Tesla's alternating current is going on here? Seems as if the brain is not only held under gunpoint by cholesterol, it is another site of production. Because of the blood brain barrier that we mentioned earlier, cholesterol cannot get through to the brain from the blood. Therefore, any cholesterol around the brain, which accounts for a decent bit of cholesterol in general, is produced on site. To top it all off, cholesterol is embedded in myelin, a substance that forms a protective sheath around axons, the parts of neurons that send messages to other neurons.

Are we all lost? Is every human being on the planet aboard the RMS Cholesterol Titanic headed for the iceberg? Not only is cholesterol around the areas where our nerves are sending information, it is also present in cell membranes, which some would say is a necessary part of the cell. We can't seem to get away from it.

This is all starting to sound like the bad plot of some made-for-TV movie with an antagonist who knows no equal and cannot be stopped. A logical individual would know that the point is that we're looking at the different types of cholesterol. There is always mention about keeping your good cholesterol up and your bad cholesterol down. Let's take a look at cholesterol itself and see if we can get to the bottom of all this from the chemical approach.

Cholesterol, Defiler of Logic

What is cholesterol? Cholesterol is cholesterol. If that sounds maddeningly simplistic and inexplicable, that's because it is. Although it is referred to frequently as a lipid, fat, or steroid, cholesterol doesn't appreciate that because it doesn't quite fit any of those descriptions. Sometimes, it is even called a combination of a steroid and alcohol, but it doesn't behave like an alcohol. It seems like cholesterol is always trying to be the rebel. Perhaps it is that the proverbial bad cholesterol is the rebel, while the good cholesterol is trying to fight the good fight.

This is where we run into a problem of classification. Perhaps it is not so much a problem, so much as a blatantly incorrect label. Basically, bad cholesterol is the term for low-density lipoproteins (LDL) while good cholesterol is the term for high-density lipoproteins (HDL). You might ask why the actual word "cholesterol" isn't in those titles. It isn't because they aren't cholesterol. They belong to the group of players who are known as variable transports for triglycerides, phospholipids, cholesterol, cholesteryl esters, and proteins. Going in order from largest to smallest, they are chylomicrons, very low-density lipoproteins (VLDL), intermediate density lipoproteins (IDL), LDL, and HDL.

While we can provide brief summaries of action, we don't want to go too much into the details and variable percentages of composition or else we'd bog down the flow. Basically, chylomicrons have the responsibility to get the cholesterol and fats from the intestines and bring it to the liver for assimilation and future use. VLDL is the next transport, and unlike chylomicrons, VLDL transport products are actually made inside the body, as opposed to those taken in by the actions of the chylomicrons. IDL are more temporary in nature and simply ferry items back to the liver.

LDL, or "bad cholesterol," is a transport of both cholesterol created within the body due to local synthesis and cholesterol taken in through diet. It is also the primary transport of cholesterol and accounts for more than 50 percent of all circulating lipids, bringing cholesterol to where it is needed. LDL is involved in the formation of those atherosclerotic plaques on artery walls that we talked about earlier. Meanwhile, HDL works like a vacuum cleaner; it sucks up any cholesterol that wasn't used by cells and brings it back to the liver. From there, the cholesterol is either re-assimilated to be reused or given the boot via bile. For individuals wanting a little bit of hard numbers regarding composition, here is a reference chart for the actual numbers (on the chart, note that an ester is a chemical compound derived from something):

	Triglycerides	Cholesterol Esters	Cholesterol	Phospholipids	Proteins
Chylomicrons	85-88%	3%	1%	8%	1-2%
VLDL	50-55%	12-15%	8-10%	18-20%	5-12%
IDL	24-30%	32-35%	8-10%	25-27%	10-12%
LDL	10-15%	37-48%	8-10%	20-28%	20-22%
HDL	3-15%	15-30%	2-10%	24-46%	55%

Something from the above table might have caught your eye. This something might have been the fact that not a single one of those transporters comes even close to a 100 percent value of cholesterol. Why is that relevant to our discussion? The terms "bad cholesterol" and "good cholesterol" imply that it is cholesterol, with no if's, and's, or but's about it. Based on those listed percentages, not a single one of those lipid transports can be simply called, or even come close to being called, "cholesterol" because it makes no sense. One might argue that based on the functions of LDL and HDL, "bad" and "good" labels are somewhat appropriate.

However, that has no bearing whatsoever on the fact that the word "cholesterol" is right there, included in the terms. This gives people who trust the industry to provide reliable information an impression that there are two types of cholesterol, and one of those types of cholesterol is out to get them. This nomenclature coupled with the huge push to lower cholesterol values gives cholesterol an overall bad name. But, of course, there is only one type of cholesterol.

Before we go further, it is prudent to note what the very popular lipid profile test includes. On first glance, one might see that the value is right there in the test: total cholesterol printed out as clear as the Mississippi River. Right below that value you will notice three to four other names: HDL, LDL, Triglycerides, and sometimes VLDL. What impact do they have on the number of your total cholesterol? According to the formula, they are your total cholesterol.

$$\text{Total Cholesterol} = \text{HDL} + \text{LDL} + \frac{Triglycerides}{5}$$

Clearly, based on our previous observation and analysis of composition, this might not be the most accurate display of cholesterol amounts. Can it give us an idea of how many transport molecules there are moving to and fro? Sure, but if cholesterol is popularly classified as a WMD, then it would be nice to see if the trucks transporting said weapons are empty, full, or maybe just one warhead shy of being half full.

HDL, LDL, and VLDL are added together to create your total cholesterol value. When triglycerides are tested, this value is divided by five to receive an estimation of the amount of VLDL. However, one might say triglycerides should not be called cholesterol because they aren't cholesterol at all. They are, in fact, an excellent method of storing excess calories that are not readily utilized after we consume them. In essence, a food that is practically fat-free but has an immense carbohydrate content can increase the production of triglycerides if you eat it in excess, which has the potential for throwing levels off without the direct involvement of cholesterol. The point of all this is that whether you are testing for the three lipoproteins or the two lipoproteins and triglycerides, you are not directly measuring the level of actual cholesterol. The label "total cholesterol" is inherently flawed because this is a test for the amount of carriers in the blood, which all have variable amounts of actual cholesterol.

You may recall that the actions of LDL and HDL were said to bring cholesterol to where it is needed, as well as that cholesterol is in the cell membranes. Now, the cell membrane surrounds all cells, thus largely constituting what defines a cell. The membranes play a large role in maintaining cell homeostatic balance, and they also let in what is needed while expelling what needs to be along on its way. Without a functional cell membrane, there is no cell of which to speak. Cholesterol is a major building block of these cell membranes. At this point, a person might, just might, say that cholesterol seems to be somewhat important to the body in certain regards.

Working Day and Night

Let's take a look at high and low cholesterol. The proper name for high cholesterol is *hypercholesterolemia*, which is associated with atherosclerosis. However, we will simply refer to it as high cholesterol because the individuals behind the name "hypercholesterolemia" did not take into consideration the movements of the tongue in trying to say that name over and over again. As we briefly mentioned earlier and will go into more detail soon, atherosclerosis is the buildup of plaque on the arteries, which contains cholesterol, among other things. Whenever high cholesterol is seen, the possibility that atherosclerosis is lurking in the bushes is of great concern to all involved.

What exactly are some of the indicators or issues that we can associate with both high and low cholesterol?

Before we begin looking at examples, let's start the game with a curveball. First, there are instances where the presence of high cholesterol is in no way malefic. What is the one thing that is most not associated with illness and death? That would be the creation of life, of course. For this example, we talk about pregnancy because there is certainly nothing malefic about a pregnant woman (though husbands going on midnight runs for Mongolian beef might disagree). What does a pregnant woman have to do with elevated cholesterol? A lot, apparently. Total cholesterol, LDL, and triglycerides all increase significantly during pregnancy, up to the seemingly coronary-narrowing amount of 314 milligrams per deciliter.[2-7]

Nobody can deny that the number we just wrote is high. However, pregnancy is something as basic as human life itself, because that is how we keep increasing our numbers. Are pregnant women falling over left and right from high cholesterol? One would say no, though decreased coordination may factor into a stumble or fall. After the child is delivered, the mother's levels of total cholesterol decrease in great measure in the next three months and then further decrease in the next nine months.[8] One might presume that this increased level is going up due to all the construction going around in the uterus since growing a new person requires a lot of new cell membranes to be formed. In fact, if overall cholesterol and LDL levels are diminished during a pregnancy, there is a bigger threat of miscarriage.[9]

Now, we are going to think outside the box; so work with us here. Let's say that there's something, anything at all will do, that in the appropriate amounts will help a woman keep a pregnancy and in decreased amounts will increase her risk of a terminated pregnancy. Would you in any way approach this thing as something "bad" or want to decrease the level of it? Unless you are an individual bent on the extermination of mankind, the answer is probably "no." Just some food for thought.

Let's keep riding the creation train a while longer and look at children. High cholesterol was found in up to 53.1 percent of school-aged children.[10-14] What an outrage. Where are all the statin drug commercials for little Timmy? Certainly, there are a lot of older people riding bikes in those advertisements. Maybe Timmy wants to get in on the action too, but how can he with high cholesterol? Perhaps, in a glorious period of illumination, logic would dictate that in such cases these higher cholesterol levels are associated with construction and growth. Sabotaging that process via artificial lowering would probably not be the best idea.

Pregnant women and children aside, there are also examples of adults in the purely building-up process. When athletes are training for sports, such as hockey or soccer, their cholesterol levels show an increase.[15] Consider this example: People who play such sports professionally are trained to endure a lot of physical punishment. Soccer players have to keep up a quick pace for long stretches of time during a game and learn how to expertly fall down so as to give opposing players yellow cards. Additionally, hockey can be a pretty violent contact sport and there are no pirouettes on this ice, only blood. Anyone who says that individuals in such sports are not fit and healthy is either a fan of the other team or hasn't seen the amount of fake teeth in the hockey leagues.

Cholesterol's Bargain with the Reaper

Let's take a brisk but not pleasant walk through cholesterol and its associations that we have in regards to people dying, which is a very important association because death is something we want to stay far away from. Let's look at the straight association, the one that all these cholesterol-lowering measures are trying to prevent—death related to heart disease. High cholesterol is a huge risk factor for atherosclerosis and myocardial infarction.[16,17] However, the major issue is that when cholesterol levels are lowered through the popular method of cholesterol-lowering drugs, the overall rate of death is not offset by the number of people not dying due to heart attack.[18,19]

Let's consider both ends of the spectrum. Both high and low cholesterol are associated with an increased risk of premature death.[20] Does that do anything for us? We have to consider that extremes of any sort can be associated with negative things. Coffee that is too hot burns our tongue and prevents us from enjoying more of that sweet caffeine, and coffee that is too cold can quickly turn into a popsicle. Extremes warrant wariness, at the least, since boiling or frozen coffee doesn't increase your risk of dying (but a cup of generic coffee might make you feel as if you'd die for a decent cup of the good stuff). Still, we wouldn't advise driving down the highway with a topless coffee mug.

For example, during hospitalization, people generally don't exactly want to pay the nightly cost of a hospital room. So, if an individual is healthy, he or she isn't going to be kicking it back and enjoying the fine selection of hospital pudding flavors. In one observation, the average cholesterol levels of hospitalized individuals who died as opposed to those who lived to fight another day were a good bit lower.[21] In this case, the difference in average levels was between 163.6 milligrams per deciliter and 217.8 milligrams per deciliter. Two things might jump out immediately from those numbers. The first is that the difference is actually pretty sizeable, and the second is that the latter number is above the normal range of 200 milligrams per deciliter. Another study of hospitalized individuals over the age of 65 showed that lower cholesterol levels were a predictor of an increased risk of death.[22] In this particular case, the level range that was most dangerous was below 160 milligrams per deciliter.

As for coronary heart disease, we know that there is a large association between cholesterol and atherosclerosis. Patients with this disease who had cholesterol levels below 160 milligrams per deciliter had the highest rate of death while those with levels above 240 milligrams per deciliter had the lowest risk of death.[23] One would expect such a result to not occur at all. Meanwhile, individuals older than 70 years with increased total cholesterol levels, low "good cholesterol," and high ratios of total cholesterol to HDL did not have an increased overall death, increased death from coronary heart disease, or hospitalization resulting from heart attacks.[24] For men, the lowest amount of overall death was observed in the range between 180 and 239 milligrams per deciliter, and decreasing it below this range resulted in increased risks from cancer and other diseases.[25]

These seem like big hits below the belt all around. First, high cholesterol doesn't appear to be nearly as big a scourge as it is made out to be, especially when speaking about the rates of death that should be the prime indicators regarding the overall danger of something. Secondly, low cholesterol actually appears to be worse off in allowing people to survive when they check in to a hospital, and survival is oddly enough the primary reason that most people become hospitalized rather than letting things "run its course." Even the old "good cholesterol" doesn't seem to be as great as they say.

In fact, if HDL gets such a good rap, being good and all, then why aren't there drugs that simply raise HDL? Actually, this was a considered option, but because of certain issues, this drug never saw the light of day. What could possibly be an issue from a drug that raises good cholesterol, one might say? During human trials of the drug, Torcetrapib, risk of death was increased by 59 percent and the risk of heart issues also increased by 25 percent. This seems really strange because it made sense on the hypothetical paper on which these things always make sense.

Let's take a deeper look at the issue and think about HDL's function. One of its jobs is to wander about the body to pick up and salvage cholesterol wherever it may be found so that it can be brought back to the liver for re-absorption. One interesting aspect of HDL is an almost chameleon-like property, and in the standard phase, it is anti-inflammatory, but during an acute phase response, it becomes pro-inflammatory. This makes the seemingly "good" become a "bad" because it increases the risk of atherosclerosis.[26]

Now, let's take it step by step with the inclusion of a drug that artificially increases HDL. In a well-balanced system, HDL is keeping the equilibrium up by returning unused cholesterol so that it can be infused back into the system. Now let's introduce a gluttonous mass of HDL without the associated increase of cholesterol. Suddenly, this pillaging horde is trying to take more cholesterol out of the system than should be taken out. If you keep picking the pepperoni off the pizza, then you'll wind up with a cheese pizza, which might not be what you were in the market for. In our case, rather than dealing with the distinct unpleasantness of having a subpar pizza, one would be more likely to die or have heart issues.

Immune Support and Revelations

Let's get away from overall death as a statistical observation for a bit, important as it is when speaking about cholesterol, and look at something that might not be thought of as cholesterol's strong point or as any point at all for that matter. We might still be looking at death, but let's look at it from the viewpoint of immune system function and the relationship that might be present between it and cholesterol. Cancer is certainly something that we can associate with impaired immune function. If we aren't talking of external factors like heavy doses of radiation, part of a cancer's possible progression is because the immune system suddenly finds that it didn't pick off that one straggler cell that won't know when to die properly and is now multiplying all over the place. The problem with this is that because we are not planted firmly in comic book lore, uncontrolled cell growth leads not to super regenerative abilities but to cancer that has the capacity to kill.

People suffering from advanced lung cancer, lymphoma, and cervical cancer had cholesterol levels that were lower in comparison to their healthy control group.[27] Low cholesterol in men was associated with higher incidences of colon and stomach cancers, as well as cancers in other locations.[28,29] There is even an inverse correlation between total cholesterol and LDL levels in association with the incidence of cancer.[30,31] Suffice it to say, that is an awful lot of cancer associated with lower cholesterol values.

Decreased cholesterol isn't only locked to cancer associations. There is also an association between decreased levels of cholesterol and increased rates of hospitalization from pneumonia and the flu for people in general, as well as increased hospitalization from chronic obstructive pulmonary disease in men.[32] The flu is a bit heavier than the common cold, and people do die from it every year. However, all in all, for a healthy individual, the potential yearly scuffle with influenza is usually a miserable affair but hardly hospital-worthy. Drinking some extra hot tea as opposed to spending time in the hospital just might be a preferable course of action for some people. As for chronic obstructive pulmonary disease, if there is one thing more annoying than having an obstructed lung function, it is being hospitalized with an obstructed lung function.

Furthermore, decreased cholesterol levels seem to be associated with changes in how the body functions when it is undergoing an inflammatory response from infections.[33] As we mentioned before, the inflammation process is your own body reacting to the invasion and being a little overzealous in its defense effort. Low cholesterol seems to be a marker for increased risk for HIV in men, and is associated with immune system impairment while infected by this virus.[34,35] We can look at this just like the influenza hospitalization, where something already not great is made worse. In this particular case, the link is perhaps even more significant because the way in which HIV works is by going to town on the immune system and has a much greater severity. One further note on the observation of hospitalized patients is that individuals who have low cholesterol prior to going under the surgical knife have a greater likelihood of the occurrence of infections post-operation.[36]

Oh Cholesterol, You Crafty Devil

All right, this is probably starting to make about as much sense as that time we got inebriated and tried to read *Crime and Punishment*. We told you cholesterol was hard to define. So, it turns out that cholesterol doesn't exactly seem to be out to get us on a widespread scale. Far from it, it actually plays a role in building up our bodies and in the creation and maturation of humans in general. It is certainly associated with total death, but almost certainly not in the way that we are used to hearing about. On top of all that, it seems to be a very good predictor of helping us fight off cancers, infections, and disease. What in the Sam Hill is going on with this sorcery?

Now, we introduce the full extent of cholesterol's power. Are we finally going to showcase the functions that make cholesterol to be the great antagonist that wants us dead? Will we finally see what crimes against humanity this molecule has concocted? Maybe not so much. We present to you, exhibit A:

The Sinister Role of Cholesterol

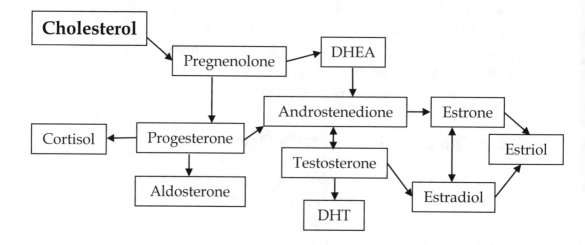

What manner of dark magic is this? What is cholesterol doing on that chart, the chart associated with steroid hormones and all the good things that they do? As it turns out, the steroid hormones are actually made from cholesterol. An enzyme hits cholesterol with several big smacks across the face and thus pregnenolone, our grandparent, is created. What follows, obviously, is that the origination of the steroid hormones comes from cholesterol.

Remember that pregnenolone has vital functions and starts the conversion to all the other steroid hormones. DHEA is found throughout the body in large quantities. Testosterone makes men what they are and keeps the brain working properly. Estrogens define women and provide a wealth of benefits in the body. Aldosterone helps regulate salt balance and has an impact on blood pressure. All these very important chemical messengers that help the human body to grow and function properly are created from public enemy numero uno.

We've said plenty about the merits of a restorative medicine approach, so how does this fit in? How does the restorative approach work with high cholesterol, and why is there such a rampant distribution of high cholesterol all over the place? If we didn't have an answer to these questions we knew you'd ask, we probably wouldn't have written them out. That would be pretty embarrassing.

The "Cholesterol is a Pretty Cool Guy" Hypothesis

Granted, we don't call it that. If you approach problems scientifically, then you have to give them boring scientific names. It's a prestigious tradition. Okay, here is the rub — our hypothesis is that steroidopenia is a result of aging and, as such, is a primary mechanism of hypercholesterolemia, which then itself is identified as a consequence of age-related, enzyme-dependent down regulation of steroid hormone biosynthesis and their interconversions. The full, scientific description goes along with its scientific name: *hormonodeficit hypothesis of hypercholesterolemia* (hooray for alliteration). See what happened there? All the fun is just magically sucked out of the room. Just right out. Close the window because there is a giant science tornado outside and all the fun is getting blown right out. Let's break that down for the benefit of what we're sure are the scant few among us who don't have an advanced, inborn comprehension of chemical and biological principles backed up by a rich knowledge of Latin.

We can knock off steroidopenia first because that's a simple one. *Penia* is from the Latin for deficiency, and steroids we don't have to explain because surely you've been paying attention this whole time. Jam those two together and what we have is literally the deficiency of steroid hormones. Hypercholesterolemia we already explained as the name for high cholesterol that we avoid saying because it isn't kind to the mouth. The term "enzyme-dependent" calls back to the little detail we mentioned about enzymes and how they are instrumental in the conversion processes between steroid hormones. "Down regulation" is simply a reference to the decrease of cellular components in response to an external variable. "Biosynthesis" is more evidence of Latin at work and refers to the conversion of products into more complex ones under the influence of enzymes.

Let's translate that into the common tongue of men: Elevated levels of cholesterol can occur when steroid hormone levels are decreased because steroid hormones are created from cholesterol through enzyme action and this function declines with age. Unfortunately, in the cutthroat world of scientific articles you have to sound just as important as everyone else who is trying to sound important, which is the reason for the wording of the actual hypothesis. But why, you might ask, the high cholesterol?

Let's look at it from the viewpoint of the body. As we might have implied before, the body can be both brilliant and dumb at the same time. Think of it as having great book smarts but the common sense sometimes gets a bit neglected. You would want an Oxford professor to help you with a bit of math, but you wouldn't necessarily want him on your side in a violent street hooligan brawl after Manchester United loses a football match. So, the body looks at steroid hormone levels in the body, and it makes some assumptions.

The main issue is that it isn't feeling too hot because all those steroid hormones are necessary for a lot of different functions, and it hasn't quite felt the same ever since they decreased and the dog ran away. Meanwhile, cholesterol is the building block of the body and is responsible for the creation of steroid hormones. At this point, the proverbial light bulb turns on above the head and the body starts to hatch a plan together. It puts on the lab coat and goggles (we really wish it wouldn't do that sometimes) and begins to add together what it knows. Hormones are normal and cholesterol is normal; all is fine in the world. Hormones are low and cholesterol is the old normal level, so then why are the hormones low? Ah, but we must make more cholesterol to make up for the deficit!

Yeah, good effort on that one, body, just somewhat misguided. As the body ages, it has trouble putting together all the hormones that it had no issues with earlier in life. So, maybe if we increase the cholesterol level, as in increase the raw material so that the finished products can be more readily assembled, then the whole low hormone thing will blow over and become normal again. Yet, as we know, the problem isn't a lack of cholesterol but a breakdown in the enzymatic action that comes about due to age.

Let's think of a city, perhaps in ancient times because, back then, an overinflated bureaucracy wasn't in charge of city planning. As the city grows to be able to support the purpose for which it was envisioned, there are ample construction supplies and workers putting everything in place, building up and maintaining all the construction. Then, slowly over time, the city begins to function at a poor level. Buildings are falling into disrepair, potholes are causing trucks laden with necessary goods to swerve off the road and crash and burn, and everything in general is just falling into a sad state. The city, in a panic, orders for more supplies to be made and delivered so that all of these problems can be fixed. Unfortunately, nobody took note of the warehouses to see that the necessary supplies are all there. Instead, it seems that there are fewer workers to take those supplies and to keep the city running smoothly. Maybe the bureaucracy was in charge of city planning after all.

An individual learned in the ways of the world and possessing many different blood tests might at this point say, again, "But my cholesterol is fine and my hormones are still low!" There is another hypothesis that we wanted to mention called Relative Hypercholesterolemia. As a quick example, let's look at two individuals, in which the levels of "high cholesterol" begin past the 200 milligrams per deciliter mark.

	25 Years old	45 Years old
Julius	140 mg/dL	170 mg/dL
Marcus	170 mg/dL	210 mg/dL
Octavius	189 mg/dL	225 mg/dL
Flavius	150 mg/dL	180 mg/dL

Here we are observing some people, Romans apparently, and how their cholesterol values changed as they aged. This is a very simple way of looking at relative high cholesterol. Julius and Flavius are doing pretty well, it seems, with both of their cholesterol values being below that dreaded 200 mark. Marcus and Octavius aren't doing as well, and any moment now, their doctors will probably tell them to lower their cholesterol. Yet, look at the overall comparison for all four people from left to right. Everyone's cholesterol levels increased, regardless of the fact that some of them wound up above the threshold or below it. Thus, what we have here is high cholesterol in that it is high relative to the point where it originally was when steroid hormone production was peak.

We must also mention the boor ruining the dinner party — low steroid hormone production due to low cholesterol levels, though this particular boor can be influenced by synthetic decreases of cholesterol. Nobody really seems to win at this one. Recall all the negative associations that we have observed with low cholesterol levels and put that into context with not enough building blocks for the production of all those steroid hormones. Things then begin to look pretty grim. Certainly grim like the world appears to the multitude of individuals with psychological disorders who have low cholesterol.

Where There's Smoke, There's Fire

Let's take a look at this relative to the definition that we can give cholesterol. Put aside the fact that cholesterol doesn't have a strict definition according to what it is and focus on how we can define cholesterol as it presents itself to the rest of the body. Consider a thermometer. You look at the thermometer and can make some pretty accurate assumptions. It gives you the ability to know if you should go outside and cook some meat on skewers in your shorts or if you should take a big swig of expensive vodka and go break the ice in the lake and swim in your underwear. The thermometer tells us what the actual temperature is outside. We can look at the value of cholesterol in our body as both a rudimentary measuring tool and the units of the actual tool.

However, the thermometer analog doesn't quite cut it with cholesterol and its unique style. When we look at a thermometer, we are asking a question: how hot or cold is it outside? The thermometer answers our question by giving us a value about the actual temperature that is outside and with very little room for error. Also, we apparently have a talking thermometer that is all the rage with kids nowadays. Now, let's think about a cholesterol blood test while taking into consideration the link between it and declining steroid hormone production. In fact, let's look at several examples.

Let's say that you get your blood test and say, "Cholesterol! Oh cholesterol! What be thine value?" Well, that cholesterol will tell you, no problem at all. Now it is up to you to interpret those numbers. Some people have values of 155, 160, and 170. Based on how we naturally look at it, we would say all those people are fine. Meanwhile, some people have levels of 230, 240, and 245. We would say that those people are not fine. We can say with a great amount of certainty that the last three have disruptions in their steroid hormone production leading to the over-compensation. Well, what about the first three? All of these individuals could potentially have low steroid hormone production because, even though their cholesterol may be within a normal range, their levels could be higher in relation to what they used to be.

A cholesterol test gives us back the cholesterol value and can possibly tell us something. This something is that because you have high cholesterol, there is a problem in the body. The key to your understanding of this is that high cholesterol is not the problem but is rather the indicator that there is a problem. Just like high cholesterol levels indicate problems, smoke is a way of telling us that something is burning. Let's think for a second and see how this applies to cholesterol-lowering drugs. Imagine, if you will, the fire brigade, but instead, they are called the smoke brigade. They don't go around putting out fires. Instead, they go around and make sure that there is no smoke anywhere. Everything is still burning, but, hey, at least we don't have any of that pesky smoke floating about right? Clearly, one might say that there are a few kinks in such an approach to the prevention of dangerous conditions.

But, again, since the body is so complex, simple analogs like this don't always cut it. Lowered hormone production has to make do with the cholesterol it is given and maybe even get a nice buffer from the elevated cholesterol to be able to keep up its steady rate. Well, what happens when cholesterol-lowering drugs are introduced into this equation and take away the cholesterol that is in this delicate and already malfunctioning system? The levels of hormones can possibly drop even further.[37] Let's consider such a situation.

Cholesterol is normal, hormones are normal, but of course then the body has to go and start breaking down. Cholesterol increases to try and make up for the lowered hormone levels, but alas, it can only do so much. Cholesterol lowering-drugs come into the picture and lower the cholesterol levels so that it looks like everything is all right. However, hormone levels are still low. But wait! There's more. The cholesterol drugs are liable to be so effective that they may even bring cholesterol down lower than it was during optimal conditions. Now, we find ourselves in quite a double whammy situation. The cholesterol level becomes lower than what the steroid hormone production requires, which can result in even lower hormone levels. On top of that, the cholesterol levels from the blood test would seem to imply everything is fine when, in fact, it is even worse. Elevated cholesterol levels are telling us that something is not fully functional in the body, and instead of addressing that problem, we are just creating the dangerous illusion that everything is fine when it is possibly even worse.

Simply recall the laundry list of side effects we discussed that can arise from the use of cholesterol-lowering drugs in Part II. Without having the proper knowledge, one might think, "Man, those are some pretty strong drugs, but at least my cholesterol is going down." Once a person is adequately aware of the cholesterol-hormone link, suddenly, the possible list of side effects can explode. On top of statin drug-specific side effects, anything that is related to a decline in hormonal levels can also potentially manifest itself as a side effect while using the conventional therapy of cholesterol-lowering drugs. We particularly noted statin drugs earlier on because of the way they work to decrease the amount of cholesterol by inhibiting an enzyme that is part of the chain towards cholesterol creation (which has the bonus side effect of impacting the links in that chain leading up to the actual cholesterol molecule).

In our own experience of blood test analysis, the lowest hormone levels for the major players are often associated with the use of cholesterol-lowering drugs. We would elaborate further on that, but after describing the situation as we have, there's really not much to say. The logical chain of events simply reinforces what we have already described. But, what about the restorative approach to solving this problem?

Our restorative approach goes hand in hand with what we have described about our program and testing protocol already. A primary force behind our approach is the restoration of steroid hormone levels to help with the issues related to them. It would stand to reason, then, that when the restoration of hormones to their optimal levels is achieved, then the elevation of cholesterol should be normalized. Is this another one of those cases of it looking solid on paper but failing in practice? Fortunately, not.

In our experience, the multi-modal approach to the restoration of hormone levels brought with it the normalization of cholesterol levels, as well. Note that we specifically mention the normalization of cholesterol and not the lowering of cholesterol. To lower cholesterol is to speak in absolutes about lowering a number that is the indicator and not the true cause. The normalization of cholesterol is achieved by approaching the problem from the logical point.

Hypotheses Need Friends Too

From a logical approach, this would all seem to make sense, but that isn't how things work around here. Leonardo da Vinci's aerial screw helicopter prototype certainly looked very nice on a piece of aged parchment, but it would never actually fly.

As good as the logical approach is, the practical approach is the one that ultimately gets results. To that effect, we have two published studies that relate some specifics about our approach: *Hormonorestorative Therapy is a Promising Method for Hypercholesterolemia Management* and *Correction of Steroidopenia as a New Method of Hypercholesterolemia Treatment*.[38,39] Let's briefly go through these with both summary and commentary to see what happened with extended explanatory comments here and there, starting with, believe it or not, the first one of the two.

Publication I

In any publication that deals with cholesterol, we certainly can't forget to mention heart disease and how many people die from it. In this case, 50 percent of deaths is that number, which isn't exactly slim pickings.[40-42] Elevation of total cholesterol is, of course, associated with increased risks of atherosclerosis and heart disease while a decreased level is associated with a reversion of atherosclerosis in patients with coronary heart disease.[43-46] In the high risk, middle-aged population, treatment of high cholesterol is the most recognized method of keeping atherosclerotic heart disease at bay. Accordingly, many pharmaceutical and treatment methods exist in both North America and Europe.[47,48] However, although the treatment does decrease atherosclerosis, there are the problems of impaired quality of life and side effects.[49,50]

"Quality of life adjusted survival' is something that, as a term, is probably not well known to many, which is a pretty grave oversight. Basically, anytime someone is undergoing medical treatment, one has to take into consideration his or her own quality of life. The easiest example is an individual undergoing treatment for something, but being afflicted so severely by the potent side effects that the user is constantly wishing that they were dead instead. You can see where this would be a problem. A doctor certainly doesn't want the patient to feel like he's going to die more from the treatment than from the disease itself.

We previously noted that recent studies show that combined androgen and estrogen therapy can decrease total cholesterol, LDL, HDL, and triglycerides. Also, DHEA supplementation alone has been observed to lower total cholesterol and LDL. Even so, other studies have failed to confirm such observations.[51-56] One important thing that must be noted here is that such studies usually focus on giving only one dose of a certain agent to the whole population without taking into account the actual goals that should be followed in restoring their hormone levels. Our study involved 112 individuals (34 male, 78 female) at an average age of 54.2 years, and all of them receiving the hormone restoration therapy as outlined in our protocols. The time of observation ranged from three months to twelve years. This, of course, included such things as cyclical nature where applicable, individualized dosing per initial results, and only bio-identical hormone use.

As far as the actual range, the youngest person was 22 and the oldest was 81. All individuals responded to the therapy with the pre-treatment cholesterol average of 252.9 milligrams per deciliter dropping down to an average of 190.7 milligrams per deciliter, an average reduction of 24.6 percent. In men, this drop was from 268.3 milligrams per deciliter down to 188.6 milligrams per deciliter (average 29.7 percent), and in women, this drop was from 246.1 milligrams per deciliter down to 191.6 milligrams per deciliter (average 23.6 percent). However, let's not speak solely in numbers. Bar graphs say it better.

All around HDL levels dropped from 62.7 milligrams per deciliter down to 50.1 milligrams per deciliter (average 20.1 percent) but still remained above that minimum lower level of the range. We certainly would not want to decrease something "good" too much, now would we? Women seem to have loaded the dice on this one because although they saw a decrease of 23.3 percent, the men only saw a decrease of 3.5 percent. Again, we cannot look at these as "decreases" but rather as normalizations. If steroid hormone levels are being optimized, there is not as much cholesterol being produced and not as much excess floating about for HDL to pick up like a police officer making the rounds at the local college on St. Patrick's Day.

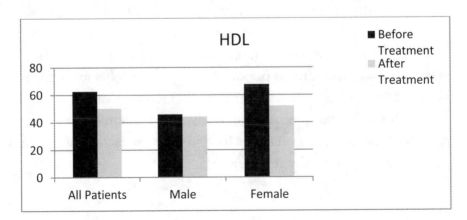

What about the proverbial bad cholesterol? We wouldn't dare forget to look at that, as well. The overall drop for LDL levels was from 154.9 milligrams per deciliter to 118.6 milligrams per deciliter (average 23.4 percent). Although the women may have won the HDL round, the men come out on top in LDL. Though, we suppose that, based on popular perception, the men kind of lose here. The drop for men was from 176 milligrams per deciliter down to 118.4 milligrams per deciliter (average 32.7 percent), and for women, it was from 148.5 milligrams per deciliter down to 118.7 milligrams per deciliter (average 20.1 percent).

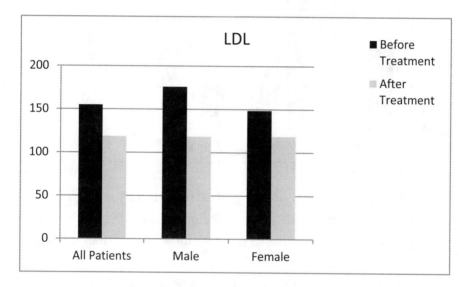

Hold on, now. We are missing a key player. That old brigand, triglyceride, which we divide by five to estimate the amount of VLDL, has to be accounted for. The overall drop was from 197.3 milligrams per deciliter down to 114.8 milligrams per deciliter (average 41.8 percent).

Men, we have good news and bad news. The good news is that you lost more. The bad news is that you lost more because your levels were breaching the stratosphere. Although women saw a drop from 144.1 milligrams per deciliter down to 104.8 milligrams per deciliter (average 27.3 percent), the men saw a drop from 348.5 milligrams per deciliter down to 143.2 milligrams per deciliter (average 58.9 percent).

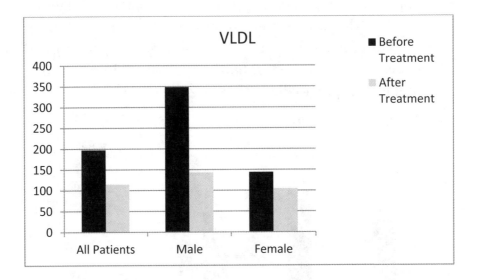

Just look at that towering structure. It almost mirrors the capacity of men to build large objects that are also very tall to penetrate the skies in order to say one message: A man built this edifice.

The problem with the human body as it ages is the breakdown of balance. No, this is not a balance that can be divined by following magnetic ley lines within the earth through the attunement of rare crystals, but rather the balance between the creative and destructive. Wow, that doesn't sound much better than the magnetic ley line thing. Basically, the human body is made to function the best it can when the internal processes that build up, termed "anabolic activity," are balanced by the internal processes that break down, termed "catabolic activity." The break down processes are not inherently bad by a long stretch because it is necessary to remove that which needs to be replaced. However, when you throw age into the equation, the problem is that the anabolic starts to get taken over by the catabolic. This normal age-related shift of metabolic activity impacts the rate at which age-associated disease progresses. Cardiovascular disease is a good example of such a disease. However, if there is a push to improve anabolic function, then the process of continuous decline can be impeded.

This needs to be kept in consideration with the overall relations of hormones and cholesterol. There is great hubbub made about the link between cholesterol and coronary heart disease, but some studies point out that individuals with "normal" levels of cholesterol experience myocardial infarctions with just as much frequency as individuals who have high cholesterol. In fact, between 45 percent and 60 percent of patients admitted to hospitals for myocardial infarction had cholesterol levels that were within the normal range.[57,58]

Our assessment of such situations is that the measurement of cholesterol increases is much more important than an absolute measurement taken at any one time. To see how high the level is in relation to previous measurements allows for an observation of the increase in cholesterol, which coincides with the decrease in steroid hormone production. This analysis can explain the occurrence of heart attacks in the absence of "high cholesterol."

Our hormone restoration approach once again uses no synthetic hormones since the latter approach is not as effective. Another key point is that this is restorative, not a replacement. "Replacement" implies a muscle-in approach with a substance that isn't what the body ordered. Restoration is just that, the rejuvenation of what the body is already producing. On the other hand, the replacement approach has the issue with synthetic hormone therapy, as well as the lack of dosing in accordance with physiologic values. This sort of rigidity on either or both counts can explain studies with controversial results regarding the use of estrogens, progestogens, androgens, and DHEA in the correction of lipid disorders.[59,60] For example, a DHEA-supplementation approach using traditional means would give the same dose to everyone to see what difference it made in lipid levels. But, what about pre-existing levels? What if the person has great DHEA levels but bad pregnenolone levels, and so on and so forth? This is why the multimodal approach has to be used to ensure useful results.

Publication II

The focus of the second study is also on the impact of hormone restoration on cholesterol levels. For our purposes here, we can look more at the levels of hormones restored because there is no information in medical literature about the connection between low steroid hormones and high cholesterol with the exception of a few studies.[61-66] Our study was an analysis of 43 individuals who underwent hormone restoration due to hypercholesterolemia. The population consisted of 12 males and 31 females. The average age was 58.4 years, 62.3 for men and 57 for women. The observation period was between three and nine months.

The protocol followed for the therapy was again the one that we described because that is what we actually use. The standards were followed for dose creation in that: recommended doses were established via clinical data and hormonal levels, individual doses were always used to bring levels to the optimal range, and the doses themselves were of the necessary amount to bring levels up to the optimal range. The use of hormones followed guidelines, as well, such as the use of only bio-identical hormones, individually modified doses, larger morning doses, hormone level tests providing adequate data, and multi-hormone therapy since a one- or two-hormone approach is inadequate in the vast majority of cases.

Below we present some hard data regarding cholesterol numbers. The average value of total cholesterol decreased from 228.8 milligrams per deciliter down to 183.7 milligrams per deciliter (average 19.7 percent). The values in women decreased from 229.2 milligrams per deciliter down to 186.3 milligrams per deciliter. The values in men decreased from 227.9 milligrams per deciliter to 177.1 milligrams per deciliter (22.3 percent).

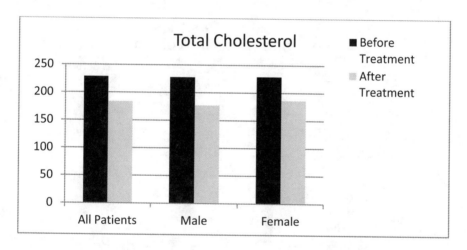

Though the sample population was of a small size, all decreases of total cholesterol were statistically significant. We mention statistically significant because if there is one thing that medical studies like to see, it is statistics. We don't want to overload on lipid test bar graphs too much, and so we will append a table of values for the players that made up the total cholesterol values.

All Values are in mg/dL	All Individuals		Women		Men	
	Before	After	Before	After	Before	After
HDL	65.0	53.8	73.3	59.5	43.6	38.8
LDL	137.4	110.2	132.8	109.3	149.3	112.5
Triglycerides	132.7	100.3	115.0	86.7	178.7	135.6

We took a gander at filling in that part of the story, and now let's look at some data from the hormone levels. Sorry, did we say no more bar graphs? We specified no more lipid bar graphs. Here are two more graphs, this time showing the difference in hormone levels before and after treatment, showing women first and men second.

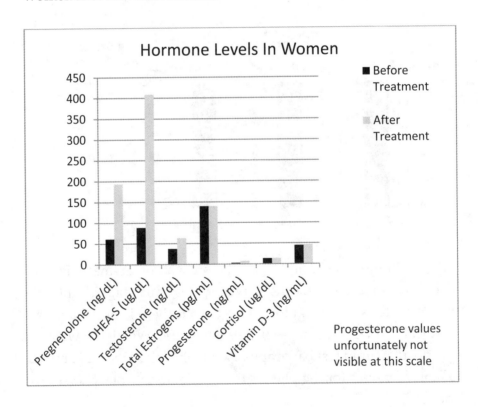

Progesterone values unfortunately not visible at this scale

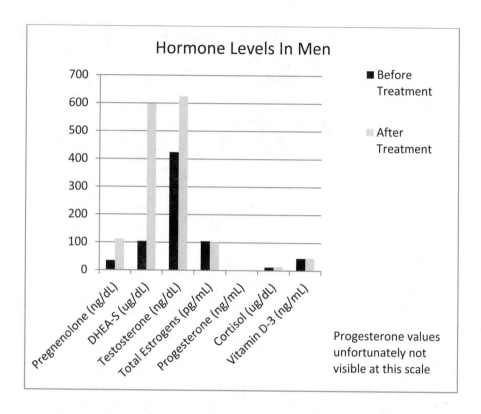

Let's talk about what this means for both genders. For men, hormone restoration lowered total cholesterol, apparently by decreasing LDL and triglycerides, but with no noticeable difference in HDL. By looking at this statement, it seems that the steroid hormones connected to the changes in LDL and cholesterol were DHEA-S, pregnenolone, testosterone and progesterone. For women, there were similar results, the total cholesterol changes accompanied by decreases in HDL, LDL, and triglycerides with significant changes in pregnenolone, DHEA-S, testosterone, progesterone. On the other hand, vitamin D-3, cortisol, and total estrogen did not have significant changes in either men or women.

Based on these observations and our knowledge of cholesterol, these results make sense. We can then follow the steps of the creation process of steroid hormones and appreciate everything that goes on. We can use this knowledge to have a second understanding of statin drugs and why they have the potential to cause the harm that they do by cutting off cholesterol production before it is even fully formed. Still, there may be one lingering question in the back of your mind regarding cholesterol and clogged arteries. We shall cover this in the very next section.

PART VI

On the Nature of Issues and Disease Related to Physiologic Breakdown

This part is to be the subject of observations and discussion of various breakdowns and diseases. However, first, we must follow through with the ending of the previous part and discuss something that we have not truly covered yet. You know to what we refer. Even now, it lurks in arteries, building up and just ready to cause problems. It is that nasty, disgusting, yellow, deposit. We just spent so much time trying to remove the tarnish from cholesterol's reputation, but was it all for naught? Is atherosclerosis going to prove us wrong and bring it all crashing down? Maybe not, and that's another one of those questions we wouldn't ask if we weren't about to do some heavy lifting. Let's take a look at the criminals, shall we?

Atherosclerosis — I Swear Officer, I Was Just in the Area

First of all, we can get one thing out of the way, a question that is always asked about this disease. What causes atherosclerosis? We don't know. That is to say, nobody knows. How can this be? After all, all those commercials, all those charts and diagrams in the doctor's offices, they all mention cholesterol.

This is the important bit that we are often too worried to notice: High cholesterol does not cause atherosclerosis. Any reputable source will make sure to specify this distinction. High cholesterol is at all times associated with atherosclerosis, but nobody can say it causes it because it does not. However, they can say that cholesterol is associated with the atherosclerotic process until the cows come home because that is a fair statement to make.

Although we do not know what causes the process to begin that leads to the buildup of atherosclerotic plaque, we do have a good picture of everything that goes into it. Basically, atherosclerosis is the body's response to an inflammation in the arterial walls via the accumulation of various components. The important bit is that cholesterol is indeed one of these components. When this response happens, LDL is the one that brings it on in to contribute to the buildup while HDL is the one that takes it out of that particular equation. This is ultimately what the terms "good cholesterol" and "bad cholesterol" are referring to, completely misguided and baseless titles as they may be. Still, the intention behind the naming can nonetheless be seen.

Iron Gut

Macrophages play an extremely large role in the initial development stages of the buildup process. "Macrophage" may not be a household name. A macrophage is a type of white blood cell, the old guard in charge of keeping our body secure against foreign threats. Although they cannot go outside the body to hunt for germs of mass destruction, they do a very fine job keeping the defensive integrity of our own body in check. The macrophage is also the big boy of the bunch, the biggest white blood cell floating about at a whopping 21 micrometers (10^{-6}). The Greeks, once again, do not disappoint, and the name is very indicative of what it does. "Macro" referring to big and phage referring to "eating." Thus, it breaks down into "big eater." With a name like that, the criminals of the seedy pathogenic underworld better watch their step as they flee in terror.

The reason that "big eater" is so apt is because it does

exactly that and does it very well. The term for this kind of behavior from this sort of fellow is called *phagocytosis*, a word when broken down from Greek (what else) roots, goes something along the lines of "the devouring cell process." We don't mean to cloud your judgment with an image of a cell going to town on a buffet, but rather a process of engulfing certain matter and then absorbing it. Instead of all-you-can-eat taco day at the college food court, imagine a giant mass slowly engulfing something until it is nothing more but ready to be broken down into the constituent parts. Clearly, it makes for a horrific and slow death for pathogens.

However, keeping the home turf clean of rabble-rousing invaders is not the only way macrophages use their big appetite to keep the body running. Recall that we mentioned that the anabolic and catabolic processes are at all times working within your body to keep things fresh. When bits of cells achieve the status of being dead rather than alive prematurely, the macrophage comes in, puts on a bib, and goes to work. There's no lobster on the menu, only necrotic tissue.

Now, it's time to note an important distinction. When cells die regularly, a chain of events makes sure to send messages to the immune system that basically says, "Man down!" Necrosis is the unexpected death of a cell, and just as the cell is about to call 911, it perishes, leaving no indication it has died. The problem with this is that such necrotic debris will decompose and release toxic substances into the body, substances that the body isn't too keen on having at the risk of grave consequences. Thus, macrophages have a crucial role in its combined task of scavenger and coroner.

Accordingly, macrophages are far from being all stomach and no brains. When the first pathogenic invaders breach the body they are liable to get eaten up, but the process here is far from a simple engulfing and subsequent break down. When the pathogen is destroyed, the macrophage acquires a chemical called an "antigen," an identifying message of sorts received from the actual pathogen, which it sends out to other parts of the immune system. When the rest of the defense force receives this antigen, it begins ramping up production of the proper defensive measures to repel the attacker. This even includes the creation of antibodies that adhere to the invaders to make further phagocytosis easier for the macrophages. In this sense, the macrophage is not only an important front line fighter but also a hybrid general helping your body to win the fight.

Eating the dead and keeping the Huns at bay are the more well-known macrophage activities, but there is also the role of creation and rebuilding. When muscle tissue is in need of repair and growth, macrophages come in with a two-wave approach. Although the first wave is in charge of putting the injured cells out to pasture to make way for new ones, the second wave helps with the regeneration effort.[1-3] Furthermore, macrophages are not solely associated with the repair of muscle tissue; their accumulation can play a potential role in the repair processes in other tissues, as well.[4]

No Alibis

What about some of the other perpetrators at the scene of the crime? We already mentioned cholesterol. Calcium is there, as well. Surely most of us know about calcium already, as most of the calcium in our body is locked up in our bones and teeth.[5] Even though it is important in areas like muscle function and nerve transmission, only about one percent of the calcium in the body is used in this way. So, what do you think it is doing at the site of atherosclerosis?

First, we must mention the process of calcification, and not the one giving you inadequate showerhead pressure. In the biological sense, calcification occurs when normally soft tissue is hardened via the accumulation of calcium. How does this apply to atherosclerosis? It occurs in the later stages of atherosclerotic buildup by taking the older, already-accumulated soft tissue and hardening it, causing it to stay in place. Although break-offs of atherosclerotic plaque are no walk in the park and can cause some serious complications, imagine if you will, what may occur during a process that hardens a buildup that has already started to block off your arteries. It's not a pretty picture and certainly is not a pretty reality. The buildup becomes more entrenched in place, which can give the rest of the plaque buildup process greater coverage to block off more blood flow. This doesn't really seem like an all-that-great function of calcium.

Other lurkers that can show up at the crime scene are thrombocytes, but most of us know them better by their common name of "platelets." They are the cell fragments floating around in the blood that are responsible for clotting functions. They also have jobs related to homeostasis and cell growth while also being carriers for various substances like ATP, calcium, and even serotonin. Of course, what we care about the most in this regard is that if we get cut by a knife-wielding football hooligan after the obsessed zealot's team lost the match, then the platelets will aggregate to the site of injury and work to stop the flow of blood. After all, we prefer for our blood to be inside of our body rather than outside.

Shooting the Messenger

Consider these components of atherosclerosis: macrophages, calcium, and platelets. If someone asked you, "Do you like calcium?" then how would you answer? Would you say, "Heck no, I hate that junk?" Odds are that you would say that, as far as minerals go, calcium is a pretty swell guy. We love calcium. We make sure the children drink milk like water so that their bones grow big and strong. We tell menopausal women to take calcium like breath mints. Everywhere you go, calcium is just great.

What about macrophages? You might not hear much about them or have forgotten them since high school biology all those many years ago, but they are very useful, as we just reminded you. You can remember back to a few minutes ago, we hope. At the very least, how could anyone react negatively to such a useful component of our immune system? Now, we can't neglect to honor platelets, Why, they're the unsung heroes of knife fighters and high-risk skateboarding teenagers. You can't call a platelet evil, and if you don't have enough of them you will bleed out pretty bad, severely throwing off that whole blood-outside-the body-to-blood-inside-the-body ratio. Well, if you must know what's bad, there's cholesterol! Man, that guy just needs to get out.

Right, we are once again dispelling misnotions and extending the bigger picture out just a bit more. We just spent a good bit of time showing that cholesterol is not only a great part of your body, it is absolutely necessary for life. Where are the similar popular suggestions to lower platelets, macrophages, or calcium levels? Yeah, they're not around. So, how is cholesterol different? It is one of the most important parts of your body yet it has such a negative reputation based on associations that these other players are just as guilty of having. Recall that cholesterol is brought to sites where it is needed for construction and creation. We don't know what causes atherosclerosis, but we can surmise that it is some kind of healing response that goes past well-meaning into "Why do you guys want to hurt me? I thought you were the good guys."

Based on our assessment of cholesterol being the unsung hero of the body and its relation to hormone production, we have a thought here. The catabolic/anabolic ratio continues to break down as we age, and there are many breakdowns that can happen. One such example is the potential for the formation of micro-abrasions in our system of blood vessels. Such miniature "wounds" should be easily healed, but, as we have seen with atherosclerosis, this doesn't quite work out because it seems like there isn't enough juice in the system to make things right.

However, recall our earlier mention of HDL functioning like a chameleon, a dirty, shape-shifting, possible saboteur. Even the assumed benefits of HDL taking cholesterol out of the atherosclerotic equation can backfire.

Now, look at all the players of the game. When you fully look at each one individually, you can't say that any are bad. Do not forget that high cholesterol is a result of impaired steroid hormone production, and so the lack of hormones certainly is not helping anything. High platelets can cause blood clots of the bad kind, and macrophages themselves can be tricked into harboring pathogens like tuberculosis. Even excess levels of calcium can cause constipation or kidney impairment. Are any of these bad as individual units based on their overall role in the body? Of course not.

Coronary Heart Disease, an Unbiased Killer

We touched on coronary heart disease earlier. We know about some of the modifiable risk factors, such as obesity, high blood pressure, smoking, physical activity, and so forth. We also know that although cholesterol-lowering drugs like statins can reduce death from the actual disease, overall death tends to stay the same. Finally, we know that surgical procedures, such as angioplasties and coronary bypasses, can provide relief, but they don't add years to the ol' lifespan.

Let's look at one of those risk factors: high cholesterol and, by extension, low hormones. We have already established that, through hormone restoration, cholesterol levels can be decreased. However, what about the actual role of hormones in this disease other than this overall normalization of cholesterol values to prevent excess cholesterol? We say this because coronary heart disease is generally thought of as a disease targeting primarily men; although this is not really the case. Cardiovascular disease is actually the leading killer of women, just as it is for men. In fact, women are at higher risk of dying from a first myocardial infarction and of having more long-term disability, as well as an even a higher risk of developing additional disease.[6,7] That last bit is also influenced by the fact that women tend to develop this disease later in life than men. Based on our quick run through of the hormones, we already saw indicators for optimal muscle function, which the heart certainly is.

Looking at testosterone as an example, in one study that followed both men and women with angina pectoris (better known as chest pain), it was shown that testosterone supplementation improved the condition for the majority of the population.[8] Another study that alternated taking a placebo with testosterone therapy showed that the therapy showed a marked improvement in angina pectoris, as well.[9] We're sure the individuals weren't all that happy while taking the placebo, what with the increased chest pain and all.

In testosterone supplementation, there is a link between actual low levels of testosterone and heart disease. The low testosterone levels compare to the severity of artery blockage in men suffering from coronary heart disease, with the indication being that high levels of testosterone can protect against atherosclerosis.[10] Such studies tend to be focused on men and tend to leave women out in the cold, but all is not lost. The various effects that testosterone has in terms of heart health is analogous to the function estrogens have in women.[11] Even testosterone supplementation itself showed improvements in women with chronic heart failure.[12] Heart failure is certainly bad enough without having the chronic adjective attached to it.

If we are looking at testosterone, we should also take a look at DHEA as far as heart health goes. DHEA converts to testosterone, and in women, provides a major source of estrogens post menopause. This action increases the appropriate protective levels in both genders. In addition to these parts of a restorative approach, is antioxidant supplements, including the common vitamins E and C, as well as the various B vitamins that have been shown to decrease risks of heart attack and even stroke.[13-22]

Andropause, the Bent Weeping Willow, and Grapefruit Prostates

Male impotency is a relatively new phenomenon that afflicts men. Anytime we look into the past, we see evidence that men were manlier. Half-naked Greeks holding the line didn't have any testosterone deficiency to speak of, clearly. Certainly, our fathers or grandfathers who fought during World War II didn't have any problems. After all, you can't take out Hitler and his Nazi minions when the soldier isn't standing at attention. Obviously, this isn't true. Male impotency may have been a part of the times, but still, the times, they are changing. Although great grandpappy was chopping down trees on the frontier and grandpa was fighting the Wehrmacht, there was no time to talk about impotence because that simply wasn't something to be talked about during the weekly man gathering and pipe smoking.

Nowadays, men are bombarded anytime they turn on the television. Commercials frequently come on speaking about the problems of male impotence and what kind of drug can help. There are even commercials now that tell men that they probably have low testosterone due to aging. "Probably" is certainly an understatement. Unless a man is an immortal Olympian (or a lobster, we suppose), then his levels will almost certainly decline.

As we have said numerous times, this is the way of nature and what happens during aging. Let's not forget flaccid details like the decrease of almost half of all androgens due to declining DHEA levels, the fact that DHEA levels can fall by up to 74 percent in the fifties, and that testosterone levels start to approach the bottom of the barrel.[23,24] In fact, 80-year-old men have about 15 percent of their original DHEA levels, and if they make it to the ripe age of 90, they will have about 5 percent left.[25] The only stiff thing most men at such an age can look forward to is a stiff neck after spending too much time on the veranda without a scarf during Autumn.

So, what about those heavily advertised, popular drugs for erectile dysfunction? Basically, they work on the concept of "if it isn't getting enough blood, fill it up." This is partly the reason there are plenty of jokes floating around in regards to how men taking such drugs can use their anatomy as a club-like weapon.

There are several physiologic links here to cover. Men who receive testosterone supplementation have increased sexual potency and viability, which is almost a given.[26] In our experience, the multimodal approach works better because testosterone is certainly not the only androgen. Here are some facts we want to throw out for your consideration: Average total cholesterol and LDL values were higher in men suffering from erectile dysfunction as opposed to those who weren't.[27,28] Furthermore, high cholesterol is associated with something men don't want to hear anything about, poor testicular function. It is also found in 65 percent of infertile men.[29] Here's the special additional bit: two classes of cholesterol-lowering drugs, the statins and fibrates, may cause erectile dysfunction.[30,31]

It's time to put on our thinking caps. High cholesterol, which, as you know, can be caused by low hormone production, is associated with erectile dysfunction. Statin drugs, which lower cholesterol values, the same cholesterol that steroid hormones are made from, may cause erectile dysfunction. Not enough testosterone naturally or not enough testosterone due to a decrease in the building block that creates testosterone may cause erectile dysfunction. If high cholesterol was the cause of erectile dysfunction, then lowered cholesterol should logically fix this problem, yes? We'll just leave it at that and talk about the other bit now.

Andropause—men might not be as familiar with it, but it is certainly happening. There is some contention about the concept of a menopause analogue in men because, although a menopausal woman loses her ability to reproduce, a male does not necessarily lose his. One could always argue that a man is only as viable in reproduction as his ability to get a soldier to stand up straight and deliver the armaments, but we digress. A major fear of aging men is the thought that the now-frequent trips to the bathroom are either from what feels like a melon-sized prostate or a cancer attacking a source of their manhood. Either scenario isn't very nice.

Prostate cancer is no friend of man or of anyone for that matter. A common notion is that testosterone can cause this situation to get outright dire, which nobody wants to happen. However, it appears that low testosterone seems to actually increase the risk of acquiring prostate cancer, and it also has an association with more aggressive prostate cancer.[32,33] Men often wish that their favorite athlete is more aggressive in their respective sport, but under no circumstances do they wish for their prostate cancer to be of the aggressive sort. High testosterone levels are associated with decreased prostate cancer risk, and high levels prior to the occurrence of prostate cancer resulted in improved survival rates.[34,35]

Menopause, the End of Monthly Visits

Menopause and andropause are the reasons we specifically titled this part with the word "issues" and not only with "disease." Certainly, men don't want to think of their erectile dysfunction as a disease, even though it is, just as we could say is the case with menopause. Again, we have to look back at the root meaning of disease and remember that it is broader than the terms of the Treaty of Tordesillas. That is to say, it covers quite a lot. It can be an infectious affliction, but it can also be anything that is a breakdown of normal conditions. We still won't call menopause a disease because it sounds a bit off, but we can certainly say that functionality is greatly impaired.

After all, not only is menopause the signaling of the end of having to worry about birth control, but it is also the time associated with everything else linked to menopause. However, of course, you, vested in the garments of basic biological know-how, understand that a major part of menopause is the major decrease in the levels of estrogens and progesterone. Let's recall our earlier description of the monthly cycle. It looks something like this:

This graph represents the monthly fluctuations of these hormones (don't pay too much heed to the numbers on the y-axis since they are there to provide a good indicator of the ups and downs of the cycle). However, when menopause moves into town, it puts a stop to this "balanced nonsense" and institutes a new rule for the ratio of estrogen and progesterone. This is what it looks like:

Certainly, you don't have to be an expert to see that this isn't so hot. It is important to note that these are ratios that are not necessarily indicative of overall numbers. Recall that our descriptions of estrogen or progesterone dominance in no way imply a large amount, just a larger amount than the other guy, or we suppose, gal, in this case. The middle marker refers to a time when a woman is not menopausal, but is nonetheless infertile because eggs are not being released. Such an issue can be brought about by chronically low progesterone. Women who have trouble conceiving and keeping early pregnancies are often given progesterone as part of the fertility treatment. As for the menopausal ratio, we can simply refer back to our deficiency and dominance charts for estrogens and progesterone.

When a woman is in her prime, things are generally going well on account of a good balance between the hormones. Then, the balance is inevitably broken. Issues can arise from the standard gallery of symptoms related to low levels of progesterone, estrogen, and estrogen dominance. We simply have to refer back to our listings to see some of the bedlam that can arise from this imbalance: fatigue, weight gain, hot flashes, hair loss, headaches and migraines, depression, uterine fibroids, fibrocystic breasts, and . . . Well, we could be here for a while listing them out. A refresher of symptoms is back in Part IV.

Postmenopausal women are certainly no stranger to hot flashes. In fact, many women experience these frustratingly hard-to-diagnose occurrences well before menopause due to the loss of the optimal hormonal balance. Nobody would deem to say that hot flashes are a mild event, lest they get punched by an angry woman who knows better, but it is certainly possible to say that in the grand scheme of things, hot flashes are not all that vile when compared to the likes of ovarian and breast cysts. These cysts, associated with low progesterone levels, are no walk in the park, and neither are cancers of the same variety.

All these issues are caused by the lack of balance, as well as the deficiency of hormones. Upkeep of this balance can have a very good prognosis on the issues that can occur due to the lack of the protective buffer afforded by both balance and higher levels. Furthermore, restoration by multimodal approach, of levels closer to the ones found earlier in life can greatly help with such nagging issues.

Migraine — Alas, Poor Brain!

You might ask why we appended this section after menopause and issues related to "female hormone" imbalance. If you have to ask this question, then you are probably a man. Unfortunately, although women get the improved life expectancy compared to men, one of the offsets is that women are afflicted by migraines with a much higher frequency. Migraines are a bit like atherosclerosis. Atherosclerosis clogs your arteries and nobody knows why, whereas migraines hurt like the Dickens and nobody knows why. That's right—science doesn't fully understand string theory and what exactly causes migraines.

However, many people are familiar with its effects, and those in the know couldn't care less about the cause in the moment. All thoughts have turned to relief. Anyone who refers to a migraine simply as a "bad headache" is probably blessed with mild migraines or has never experienced one, and we would lean towards the latter reason. Many migraine sufferers experience various indicators that signal the onset of a migraine and even have to stay away from certain dietary triggers. The only thing worse than getting a migraine is not being able to eat New York cheesecake because it can set the migraine off. More than a few individuals even get what is termed an "aura" shortly before the onset of migraine. Unfortunately, getting an aura refers not to the procurement of mystical powers but instead to visual events or impairments ranging from bright, flashing, white or multi-colored lights, blurred vision, and even zigzagging patterns across the field of vision.

Actual migraine pain ranges from severe to having the brain feel like Julius Caesar after realizing he was surrounded not by friends but dirty conspirators. On top of these murderous pains, several associated events can occur, such as nausea (a very common side event), diarrhea, or blurred vision. Another very common side effect, which can last for quite a bit, is sensitivity to light and sound, which is why many migraine sufferers retreat to a dark room and lie down. The lying down part is because a migraine is also often debilitating because, clearly, all the other issues weren't already enough. For people who suffer severe chronic migraines, the combination of all these issues can modify existing calendars, not based on 28 to 31 days, but rather on days split down the middle between functional days and "I feel like a vampire lying on the couch in a dark room the whole time" days.

All that aside, here are some very interesting parts— interesting from a scientific standpoint, of course, not in the amount of grief they cause the sufferer. A big "migraine risk factor" is menstruation.[36] Another interesting bit is that although boys and girls suffer about the same rates of migraines pre-puberty, after the fact, the ratio starts to become predominantly "in favor" of women, a bias we know and hate. In fact, migraine occurrence and overall patterns are influenced by factors like the first menstruation that a woman experiences in her life, the use of oral contraceptives (laden with hormones, of course), pregnancy, perimenopause, and menopause.[37]

Where is the common thread in all these things? It is in the fluctuating levels of progesterone and estrogens, as if we haven't thrown enough charts at you to reinforce that fact already. This is where the restorative approach comes in. Although we can't say definitively what precisely causes migraines, the same as everyone else can't say, we can certainly say a large part of it seems to be around an imbalance of various physiologic factors. This is based on our own experience with women afflicted with migraines who are on the restorative program.

What we have to stress here is that simply trying to optimize the levels and the balance of progesterone and estrogens is not nearly enough. Although they seem to play a large role in the overall equation, the use of all the hormones, such as pregnenolone, DHEA, and even testosterone, have been shown to be variably effective across different individuals. The greatest asset of the physiologic approach is also the greatest challenge: no two individuals react the same way because no two people's bodies break down in the same way. Although the overall approach works in many cases and shows great promise, it has to first reach that point by starting out on a semi-common ground and then narrowing down the specifics.

Other factors seem to play into the treatment of migraines, as well. A pretty significant one at times is the use of magnesium and the optimization of the balance between magnesium and calcium. Adequate levels of important neurotransmitters, such as serotonin and melatonin, can also play a large role. Even the restoration of impaired intestinal flora seems to play a role in certain cases, as well as does a preliminary parasitic cleanse to flush out potential infestation. Clearly, the last thing we need in our bodies is parasitic worms defecating in our homeostatic establishment.

When that perfect assemblage of agents is collected from the individualized approach along with a good dose of that old brigand, trial and error, migraines are often greatly decreased in severity or even altogether gone. In the interim, even particularly painful and long-lasting migraine episodes can be controlled by an extra addition of the items already used, the proverbial restorative torch in the woods at night against the migraine wolves.

Fibromyalgia, Not Pleasurable in the Least Bit

Fibromyalgia is another one of those fiendish afflictions targeting mostly women and having no straight, known cause, just like migraine. Although migraine affects women in a 3:1 ratio compared to men, fibromyalgia hits harder with a ratio of 9:1.[38,39] Fibromyalgia can basically be described as chronic and widespread pain, and the extra salt in the wound is that stimuli that previously did not cause pain can do so.

Let's look at some associations and how they can factor into the restorative approach. A hypothesis is floating about that fibromyalgia may be due to an irregular disturbance of the neural, immune, and endocrine systems.[40] The endocrine system is responsible for hormone production, the neural system is obviously in charge of the nerves, in which hormones play their roles, and the immune system, which can also be impacted in large part by hormones. This is a hypothesis that we can throw our hats off to because, fundamentally, it appears to make sense since our experience with the restorative approach has been used to help women suffering from fibromyalgia.

Fibromyalgia has been associated with a delayed onset of menstruation for girls and with infertility in women, both of which we can associate with hormonal imbalance.[41] Fibromyalgia sufferers have symptoms like fatigue, poor sleep, and psychological problems, which can be associated with hormonal deficiency.[42] Disorders such as migraines, panic disorders, irritable bowel syndrome, chronic fatigue syndrome, and major depression occur frequently with fibromyalgia, which seems to imply an underlying connection.[43] Furthermore, these resulting disorders and related conditions exhibit common patterns across a variety of systems.[44-47] Let's finish this one off strong and mention that a possible cause of fibromyalgia appears to be an overly excited central nervous system.[48]

Now, we may weave a complex web with our narration, and rightly so since there is nothing simplistic about our bodies, but hopefully it all links back to the center in your mind. Kind of like the link to that website we mentioned earlier in the introduction, or even that phone number at the introduction and epilogue.

Think back to our earlier discussions —anytime a steroid hormone is known for one thing, it winds up either being a neurosteroid or having very beneficial action towards neural action. Recall that a primary function of neurosteroids is to control how excitable neurons can be. Finally, we can mention the straight-up neurotransmitters in their apparent roles with fibromyalgia. The disease is associated with inadequate "deep sleep" and sleep that doesn't do its proper job of leaving one feeling refreshed.[49,50] Sufferers have been observed to have low melatonin levels. The supplementation of melatonin for individuals with fibromyalgia resulted in reduced pain, sleep issues, and depression.[51]

Relating to Afflictions of the Joints and Bone

Let's talk about arthritis, or more specifically rheumatoid arthritis and osteoarthritis. While we are here, we might as well throw in osteoporosis, even though it isn't quite in the same ballpark. On the subject of arthritis, most of us are familiar with it, if not personally then probably by knowing at least one individual who has it. As a basic definition, we can call arthritis an inflammatory disorder relating to the joints. The ones we just specified are certainly not the only ones out there, just the ones we will be mentioning here because there are over 100 different types of arthritis. Let's talk about rheumatoid arthritis first, and because that is a pain to write out and to say each time, we will call it RA.

First of all, RA is a long-term inflammatory disorder that affects not only the flexible joints, but other organs, as well. Recall our earlier discussion about the immune system meaning well but being a bit overeager in its function, leading to inflammation. RA is like the poster child of that impulsive heedlessness. What begins as a short trip down Inflammation Avenue eventually leads to buying permanent living quarters in Joint Immobility and Deformity City (what a terrible name for a town). Other unpleasant occurrences include: the growth of nodules on the skin, rheumatoid lung disease, and kidney damage.[52,53] Cherries on top of the autoimmune cake (for it wants to celebrate all its good, hard work) include high risks for atherosclerosis, myocardial infarction, and stroke, as well as an increased risk of lymphoma.[54-57]

Seeing as how RA is primarily an autoimmune disease, optimized physiologic function can certainly benefit here. Various steroid hormones work on the immune system to provide the best functionality and defense, as well as modulating the severity and fervor of response. Individuals on the restorative program can have both improved symptoms and functionality in consideration of the point of the RA's progression, which may be an impediment.

What of osteoarthritis? This one is the most common form of arthritis and is the age-related, wear-and-tear format that is also the most common form of chronic disability in the United States.[58,59] Basically, imagine if you will, all the joints and the bones they connect in your body. Now imagine said joints wearing away through the reduction of the actual cartilage, as well as the degradation of the end points of the attached bones. The concept of bones grinding on bones is perhaps more painful to think about than recalling what nails going down a chalkboard sound like.

The common conception of its cause is simply the "you're getting old" excuse, along with other factors like a long life full of regular extraneous use of the joints, being overweight, or having injuries. We certainly can't disagree with this, but can't help but notice that this isn't the whole picture here. What happens during aging? A decrease of hormones, of course, as if we haven't mentioned that enough yet. Certain hormones, such as testosterone and estrogens, play essential roles in bone health. Estrogens alone are a big factor in the balanced ratio of bone-breakdown to bone-buildup, and are responsible for keeping adequate amounts of collagen present in the human body — collagen being a primary building block of cartilage. As for the bone itself, don't neglect to remember that the end points of the bone also become worn out, and so the integrity of the bone structure is compromised, as well.

With this in mind, we piggyback onto osteoporosis and find that we don't actually have much to say. When we spoke about estrogens and the associated hormonal benefits, we covered the destructive and creative processes of bone. Throwing calcium at the problem is only half the battle and, as a single mode approach, is not necessarily the best way to go about it. A big part of osteoporosis in the view of the restorative approach is, as always, the preventative aspect. If estrogens and other steroid hormones are maintained, the likelihood of an imbalanced buildup and destruction ratio are greatly reduced.

Macular Degeneration, Ocular Occlusion

Macular degeneration is better known as Age-Related Macular Degeneration, which is then further better known by its acronym: AMD. It is also the number one cause of blindness in older adults. Without delving too far into the medical nitty-gritty of it all, macular degeneration is the degeneration of the macula (we know what you're thinking; it was a surprise to us, as well). The macula, a part of the retina, contains a large concentration of cells that can convert oncoming light into signals, thus playing a large part in our high resolution, colored vision. Therefore, functionality loss may range from blurred vision to a loss of central vision, or other impairments, such as shadows and trouble discerning contrasts. The problem here is that, unlike poor vision, putting on a pair of glasses won't help.

Macular degeneration can be further subdivided into dry and wet forms. If you think that doesn't sound very "sciencey" (yes, scientists are allowed to make up words; they're just usually long and not in English), then you would be correct. The dry variant refers to central geographic atrophy while the wet form refers to neovascular or exudative macular degeneration. Dry and wet don't sound too bad now, do they? Basically, dry refers to the atrophy of cells under the retina, leading to vision loss, and wet refers to abnormal blood vessel growth, which can ultimately leak (we apologize for that mental image) and cause damage to the light-catching cells and even serious vision loss if untreated. Dry can, in fact, transform into wet; although this is not common.

Enter drusen. These oddly named accumulations begin to, you guessed it, accumulate in the macula during macular degeneration and are composed in part of cholesterol. If you thought, "Why, what is that handsome devil doing here? Is he on a noble mission of restoration and rebuilding? I was looking forward to seeing him again," then we would raise our hands in expectation of a slow-motion high-five.

Although improvements linked to slowing down or to stopping macular degeneration (perhaps even reversing) via the restoration of steroid hormones do already look promising, macular degeneration is a bit of a slow mover, and this will take time to properly observe. A particularly good complementary and already recognized beneficial treatment strategy is the use of various nutrients and antioxidants. There is already a large amount of carotenoids in the macula, as well.

Stem Cells and Hormones, a Bold Alliance

More like, a necessary alliance. Due to media attention, we are certain that most people are at least familiar with stem cells, and so we will simply define them as progenitor cells that can turn into whatever cells the body requires. It is an all-in-one cell that has both the means and the blueprints to become whatever it needs to become. One would say that it is a useful cell, indeed. We won't dwell on the commotion associated with stem cell therapy and leave that to the politicians and activists. Specifically from our point of reference here, we will be speaking in regards to stem cells harvested from your own body.

To begin, stem cells can function so as to rejuvenate and repair the body, which can be greatly aided by well-functioning metabolic activity. What has great control over metabolic activity? Hormones. Our reasoning is that for stem cell therapy to be optimal on all fronts, optimized hormones must also follow or already be present.

Regarding the link between hormone and stem cells, first, we should mention the big players in all this: bone marrow stem cells. Studies show that stem cells from bone marrow can become cells as varied as neurons, cardiac muscle cells, skeletal muscle cells, and even the cells that line our blood vessels.[60-62] As is easily evident from this variety, stem cells can do quite a bit in restoring the functional body.

DHEA leads the charge with benefits like increasing the growth rate of human neural stem cells and the proliferation of progenitor cells.[63,64] Progesterone has many receptors in certain types of stem cells and is a key player in the defense and upkeep of the nervous system and spinal cord.[65-68] Testosterone has the potential to increase progenitor cells in the bone marrow and induces and furthers the differentiation of embryonic tissue.[69,70]

Suffice it to say, there is plenty to be said between the major controllers in our bodies and these cells that can become what we need most.

We bring this up because, although stem cell therapy is an extremely promising field in concept and already in practice, side effects from the transplants can occur. Such issues include: lowered hormone levels, such as with testosterone and estrogens, impaired menstrual cycles, and adrenal insufficiency. Stem cell therapy also currently has co-treatment regimens, which include steroids and other such pre- and post- plans, the side effects of which can be alleviated with hormone restoration.

Regarding Other Villains at the Breakdown Theatre

Here we will mention in passing certain impairments or diseases in which we can associate or potentially associate improvements based on the restorative, physiologic approach. The brevity inherent here is primarily because it is simply a refresher of what we have already mentioned previously within the context of restorative medicine.

Of Madness and Melancholy

"Madness" is perhaps a very strong word to use here, but one can never underestimate the impact that an optimized physiology can have in staving off what might seem like unlikely issues. After all, we should remember that low cholesterol is associated with violent crime, of all things.[71] Throughout this narrative we have been reinforcing the fact that steroid hormones have many functions associated with the neural realm and the proper function therein. Recall that impaired steroid hormone levels are associated with anything from anxiety disorders to depression while optimal levels or supplementation seem awash with benefits. Even Parkinson's, a serious neural impairment, is affected by hormones. We can certainly never forget the link between low cholesterol levels and suicidal tendencies either.[72,73]

Insomnia, Land of 1,000 Tosses and Turns

The causes of insomnia are far and varied. We might be worried about that meeting tomorrow, if we are going to purge our bowels tomorrow after eating at that roadside taco stand for dinner, or perhaps we are too occupied with concerning ourselves with rising gas prices. Counting sheep is hard to do when we can't afford to fill up our tank to go to the pasture. However, outside of worry-induced insomnia, there are a lot of associated physiologic factors, such as fibromyalgia, migraines, and psychological issues. A good balance of important neurotransmitters and hormones can help with this potentially serious issue, be it purely mental on our part or due to deep physiologic issues. We mustn't neglect to mention melatonin again, the neurotransmitter that is basically in charge of our biological clock.

Type II Diabetes—What Kind of Sick Person Baked All These Delicious Cookies?

Diabetes is certainly not only about being sadly barred from all manner of confectionary delights. Nobody is going to be thinking about a lack of cake-eating when poor circulation leads to the amputation of a beloved body part. On further thought, all body parts are beloved when considered in the context of amputation. Physiologic optimization is a complex process with many functions and key players, a major component of which is, of course, hormones. As far as the link with hormones, remember the big picture of hormones as metabolic controllers. Low testosterone levels have been observed in men with type 2 diabetes and are associated with increased insulin resistance.[74-76] Insulin resistance is the one resistance you don't want to build up because that is part of the diabetes playbook. Furthermore, testosterone supplementation has actually been shown to decrease insulin resistance.[77]

One bit of word play that can sometimes trip people up is the "improvement of insulin resistance." The improvement of insulin resistance is the decrease of the resistance, not the increase. Like with temptation, as they say, we may resist anything but insulin. Insulin resistance should ideally be futile. Another of the hormones, progesterone, plays an important role in the release of insulin and in the function of the pancreas (where insulin is produced, believe it or not).[78]

No, I Prefer Being Bald, and I Love Hats

Although some men look like action heroes and grizzled gladiatorial pit fighters when they go bald and shave off the rest, many other men would rather not part with their hair, thank you very much. We've already established that increased DHT is the body's well-meaning effort to make up for its decreased testosterone. The irony is lost on the body that by trying to increase the potency of testosterone function in men, it is hampering efforts at improving reproductive viability at the local bar. Cortisol would like to remind us that it too can play a hand in this with chronically low or high levels.

Our Intimate Intestinal Friends

Surely, we remember that a proper amount of the beneficial bacteria that populate our intestines is essential to our good health. The bulk of the serotonin present in the body resides here, and even issues like irritable bowel syndrome appear linked through biological cahoots with the likes of migraines and fibromyalgia. Indeed, the connections to our nervous system and our digestive system are many. This may sound like a silly notion, but recall the last time you tried to do anything on an empty stomach. Yeah, that stomach isn't going to have any of that and will make sure that you are well aware that the mighty glutton requires sustenance before he lets the brain do any serious thinking. Take note that a healthy digestive system is key to a healthy body, and on that note, we can move on to the final part.

When Bacchus isn't gorging himself on fine wines and foods, he probably isn't worrying about his cholesterol.

PART VII

On the Nature of Nutrition and Health

Nutritionist, hedge wizards, celebrities losing weight on the television, diet aids . . . One might go a bit insane trying to keep track of all the "healthy" eating and weight-loss advice to which we are constantly subjected. There is certainly enough of it floating about there. Where does weight loss and diet fit into the restorative approach? We have certainly spoken about obesity as a risk factor in a great multitude of ailments, but we haven't specifically spoken in regards to how restorative medicine seeks to make us lose excess weight.

First of all, weight loss must be approached from many directions. One could say that the battle against obesity is as multimodal as restorative medicine itself. Let's consider, for a second, our greatest enemy — fat. We go to great lengths to mention how the body does not particularly like to create things that are bad for it, but it just might happen here and there if there are breakdowns in functions. Fat is an excellent asset within our body. It helps us dissolve vitamins that are only soluble in fat and would thus be unavailable to us if it wasn't for our weight-bearing friend, fat. Yes, we called fat our greatest enemy and then called fat our friend. We hope you are no longer surprised by such seeming paradoxes.

Furthermore, fat is rather gifted in serving as an exceptional storage unit for calories, setting aside excess so that it may be employed for possible future lean times. It is even a buffer against disease, keeping us healthy longer and giving us an edge in the fight against foreign invaders. That's all great and all, but we also can't let go of the fact that our fat is keeping us out of our stylish skinny jeans. Okay, much to its offense, after all, it does watch out for us so that we don't starve, here is how we get rid of it:

First, the restorative approach seeks to make sure that everything is working in fine order. Recall how the balance between progesterone and estrogens can help with fat accumulation. Think back to how testosterone helps to build muscle and to keep fat content down. DHEA is increased with exercise and is just the little engine that can do everything it wants to because, boy, is it powerful. However, is this supremely optimized body, checked up and good to go, going to lose all your excess weight? Yes, but also no. That's a big, obese, resounding no.

Everyone to Blame

Think back to your last outing amongst the general populace. Depending on if you live in Colorado or Mississippi and the population of your locale, odds are that you saw some obese children, maybe some obese teenagers, and perhaps even some obese 20-to-30 year olds. If you think through the context of the restorative approach and all that you have found out about optimized steroid hormones and how well the body metabolism works at a younger age, you might think, 'What in the world is going on here? Aren't all these fine specimens of youth and vitality supposed to look great?'

Of course, they're not. An individual is going to look as physically fit as he or she decides to actually be. In our modern, westernized society, we have many scientific advances, perhaps one of the most convenient being the drive-thru fast food joint. We aren't even remotely going to implicate ourselves as a fast food nation chained to our delicious burger overlords. Is fast food by nature and widespread practice unhealthy? Yes it is. Should they always have healthier menu options and alternate choices? Sure, if they want to. However, is anyone holding a gun to anyone's head to go to said fast food places? We certainly hope not because that would make for a very strange kidnapping.

Okay, so fast food places are a given as a generally unhealthy choice of eating. What about restaurants? Surely, there is a wide enough variety there. Why, there are even ones tailored for the health-minded individual, serving up all sorts of foods ranging from delicious to maybe-edible, depending on the locale and one's inclination. Oh, but those portions. The value for a great meal in the United States and in many other countries approaches astronomical values in many eateries. You might pay in the range of 11 to 20 dollars and get a heaping portion of food masterfully prepared to satisfy all our darkest desires for great food. Is it going to be good? Most certainly. Is it going to be too much? Yeah, pretty much.

This is one of the biggest issues in weight gain because it is so insidious. We don't even have to specifically consider restaurants, but do because they typically up the ante. If we go out for a nice meal, our psychology is going to want to hoard that meal and finish it to the bone. We don't need doggy bags for our leftovers, for we went out for a good cooked meal and we're going to enjoy it. We are out of our home, we procured a delicious meal prepared by someone else, and our brains are going to tell us go for it. Our hunter and gatherer ancestors will be proud. Unfortunately, this type of mentality starts to transfer into other parts of our life.

Take a nice meal that, for all practical intents and purposes, we can define as "healthy." Now, make it into a heaping portion. The food is still healthy and good, but that extra portion is what truly kills it. It doesn't matter how healthy it is; if we become full or get approximately all the calories our body needs at the time, all the leftovers are going to get stored in the best way possible: fat. For the sake of our beloved and long-unworn, stylish skinny jeans, this is probably something that we want to avoid.

So, do we suggest any sort of diets as part of the restorative

approach? No. "Diet" is from the Greek word, *diaita*, which doesn't mean an altered way of eating. *Diaita* means a way of life. Our lifestyle is healthy overall, rather than eliminating choice "problem" foods from our daily gastronomic intake. This means not only choosing whether we eat the carrot or that delicious double-stacked burger, but also deciding how much physical activity we do, as well as how healthy we live our lives. The human palate is as varied as can be, and eating habits of individuals are vastly different. It is up to the individual to take on the responsibility to eat less as needed and to not making bad calls like that amazing double burger with all those extra sides or like that delicious cheese cake from the nearest grocery store bakery (hey, whatever, each small slice is only 500 calories).

The change to a healthy way of life is a big part of losing weight in conjunction with the restorative approach. Although we can't attest that a carrot could win in a no-holds, barred street fight, it certainly wins in nutritional value.

If we optimize our hormones and then don't change our eating habits, then why should we expect to lose any weight? We can't. Our body is a master at watching out for itself (remember to thank the fat for its kind and caring nature). If we uphold the status quo in dietary intake, then the body will take it as a green light to not do anything but keep that excellent emergency store of fat in reserve for us. This is the part where the other bit starts to come into play: physical activity.

Who Says Leg Warmers Went Out of Style?

We didn't just mention that dreaded physical activity to leave it at that. We always strive to help you see the whole picture, and that means we need to talk about your body's health in all aspects, including exercise and fitness. Let's get moving.

When our body demands that we get up off the couch and away from our Ngorongoro Crater wildlife marathons on the television, it's because we need to move around. It's the impetus to not let our gym membership go to waste on account of only two out of 28 days used this past February. Caloric reduction can be slow, and so exercise has to be increased to help pick up the slack. Although many might blame sedentary behavior on the American lifestyle, many people seem to lack perspective.

Imagine the old world, as it were, the old Europe, and all that good stuff. Now imagine millennia and centuries of dirty barbarians fighting over land, then some slightly more enlightened barbarians establishing castles and cities here and there, and then some more fighting but at the core that was built up from the initial forays. It is an era of horses, oxen, and peasants. Countless towns and cities grew from a very early start, the ancient age of places where people continue to build and live. This layout helped facilitate a "walking distance" thought process. As technology improved, public transportation plugged up the holes, yet many things remained within walking distance. Meanwhile, in America, things were different.

The planning of a majority of American cities outside the New England metropolitan area was done with distance and space in mind. Happy go lucky Swedes biking in their mild weather then had to spend only a couple of days traveling 15 miles to the closest grocery store in Mississippi in the summer, where breathing is akin to having a wet rag over the mouth and nose while heatstroke lurks by every magnolia tree. With similar spacial distances widespread across the country, we can see what is behind the dilemma that we face: convenience and comfort over a natural way of life involving physical exercise to commute. You might say, "But what about all those countries near the equator with all those skinny people?" First, we would mention that the nation of Kuwait is actually more obese than America, and one would certainly say it gets quite hot there.[1]

That's the point—we can't blame the weather or large distances making car travel necessary outside of certain metropolitan areas, or even the sweet, blessed air conditioning for our wave of obesity. We aren't saying that we should start biking because that's ridiculous; how are we supposed to fit all those groceries and snack cakes we bought on the back of a bike? The overall point is that any physical activity is better than no physical activity.

That is all that we recommend when it comes to achieving weight loss. The optimization of physiologic function can certainly improve energy and vigor, also known as that which is necessary to allow us to not die in the gym, but that is only 25 percent of the equation. The rest has to be filled in by each individual according to his or her abilities. We can only suggest these non-specific bits of advice in regards to losing and keeping off weight because the specifics are completely up to each person.

Anyone taking the restorative approach needs to watch out for something else. Improvement of metabolic activity relates to the optimization of the anabolic and the catabolic processes. This optimization can potentially mean that the body is up to its old tricks and is better compartmentalizing the food that we eat. Optimized intestinal flora may better access those calories it had been missing out on. Additionally, the adrenal hormones can push the body into creation mode, but without any coinciding activity, the extra effort can go into squirreling away food again. Body, you should really stop while you're ahead.

Eating Our Greens (and Oranges)

As children, we are told to eat our vegetables. As adults, we are told by people who look more fit than we do that we have to eat healthy. What exactly does that mean? Why are we encouraged to eat our "greens" and all that other "good" food when there is so much steak out there to be consumed? Besides, the cows eat the greens, we eat the cows, and everything is good right? If it were only so. What we will not be doing now is providing specific eating advice because we know no one likes to be told what to do. Instead, we will provide some illumination on what it really means to eat healthy.

If questioned, many individuals who suggest to others that they eat healthy will simply respond that to eat healthy is to eat healthy, "What do you mean what do I mean?" At this point, many would be tempted to punch the person. After all, the person was claiming nutritionist status, if not in words, then by tone, and we know that doctors are not often nutritionists and so we were really anticipating this person's good advice. Thankfully, we are going to help you understand healthy eating.

So, what is it that makes that cauliflower good or that carrot beneficial? Again, we aren't going to tell you what to eat. You're welcome. We know you're brilliant enough to know that the 500-calorie-a-slice cheesecake is not the wisest option. What we will do is run through a brief list of vitamins, what they can do, some examples of where they can be found in good quantities, and exactly why they are important based on their functional role within the body. This is also not meant to be an exhaustive list, simply one displaying some of the benefits of what is in actual healthy foods as opposed to those fabled and misbranded "healthy" foods.

Antioxidants, Defending Us From What Makes Us Live

That might certainly be a strange title, but such is the nature of antioxidants. We hear about these all the time, and that they're good for us, but what exactly are they? This is one instance where we can turn to the English language, and not the Greek, to help us out. If you are reading this, then you already know what "anti" means. Great, that's covered. An "oxidant" is referring to something that oxidizes. Therefore, an antioxidant is naturally something that prevents the oxidation of another molecule. Let's go further in depth with that.

An oxidation reaction can release free radicals, and these molecules can wreak havoc on cells. So, why do we have these oxidation reactions? It's because we breathe in oxygen. Unless you are an obligate anaerobe (congratulations on your literacy, by the way), then you need to breathe in oxygen to live. An easy example of oxygen is in the electron transport chain, which is how we get our energy. Without oxygen, we don't just lose function, we lose life.

However, because oxygen is so reactive (if there is nothing to bind to it, then it binds to itself in the form of O_2), it can cause unwanted damage to our cellular structure, including even those of proteins, lipids, and DNA.[2] We know DNA as the keeper of our genetic material, and we certainly don't want that to be damaged. Basically, antioxidants fight the good fight by preventing the oxidant from getting out of hand and roughhousing around in our body. Unfortunately for the antioxidant, this means that it itself gets oxidized. Well, at least it isn't us. We salute you, brave antioxidant. Now go die for your motherland. For our purposes here, we won't mention common foods in which you can find antioxidants for two reasons: The body produces antioxidants on its own like uric acid, and we certainly wouldn't advocate cannibalism. Secondly, some of the major dietary antioxidants are vitamins, which we will be looking at next anyway, as well as noting the foods that contain them. Therefore, we will save it for that section, thereby reducing redundancy.

Where to find antioxidants: Vitamins E and C, Beta Carotene, Ubiquinol, Zinc, Selenium.

Vitamin A

When we talk about vitamin A in foods, we are speaking about either retinol, which is the vitamin A found in the animals we eat, or carotenes, which are mostly found in the plants we eat. One particularly recognized role of vitamin A is in regards to vision, to which it is vital. Retinal (not retinol) is the form of vitamin A that allows us to see. As you can see, it is somewhat important. Additionally, it has important functions in skin health and can help with issues such as acne, psoriasis, and skin cancer.[3] Furthermore, it regulates the immune system and can even help keep out viruses and bacteria by making the skin and mucous membrane better barriers against those party crashers.[4-8]

Deficiency of vitamin A might certainly lead to vision impairment. The reason is that the deficiency can make it hard or impossible to see in low light (night blindness) and can lead to damage in the cornea and retina, which can contribute to blindness.[9] Naturally, since vitamin A is vital to the immune system, a deficiency can lead to serious issues. For example, the ability to combat infection may be impaired and result in death due to complications, such as from infectious disease in children.[10] As another example, the lack of adequate vitamin A can lead to more instances of pneumonia due to the impaired cells that line the lungs.

Decreased vitamin A levels that do not necessarily always cause outward symptoms can, nonetheless, lead to childhood issues, such as increased infections, decreased growth and slow bone development, as well as increased chance of death from serious illness.[11,12] One important thing to note about vitamin A deficiency is that outside of inadequate dietary intake, excessive alcohol consumption can deplete vitamin A levels.

Where to find vitamin A: Livers, sweet potatoes, carrots (carotenoids, anyone?), butter, spinach, pumpkin, cheddar cheese, eggs, apricots, mangoes, peas, cantaloupe, peppers, broccoli.

B Vitamins

There is a decent amount of different B vitamins around the street, and so for our run-through here we will focus on three specific ones: B12 (cobalamin), B9 (folate), and B6 (pyridoxine). Of those three, B9 is the one that is practically never referred to as B9 but rather as a folate or as folic acid. Let's take a tour of some benefits associated with these B vitamins and the dangers of deficiency.

Vitamin B12 is a bit of a hard hitter and has functions in the formation of red blood cells, proper neural function, and the creation of DNA.[13-17] Vitamin B6 has a part in a large amount of enzymatic reactions, aids in the creation of neurotransmitters, functions in sugar creation, and has its fingers in the immune system pie.[17,18] Folate has a large role in decreasing birth defects, as it is essential for the production and maintenance of new cells, as well as being required in order to make both RNA and DNA.[19]

Deficiencies of vitamin B12 can range from numbness of feet to confusion, dementia, depression, and our personal favorite—a sore tongue.[20] Vitamin B6 deficiency can lead to irritability and seizures in infants, and for everyone in general, decreased immune function and depression.[17,21] Other than the aforementioned birth defects, low levels of folate seem to be associated with increased risks of cancers, such as breast, pancreatic, and colon cancers.[22-24]

Where to find B vitamins:
B12—Clams, liver, trout, salmon, tuna, beef, cheese, yogurt, milk, ham, eggs.
B9—Beef liver, lentils, spinach, egg noodles, asparagus, macaroni, rice.
B6—Chickpeas, beef liver, tuna, salmon, chicken breast, potatoes, turkey, bananas, squash, cottage cheese.

Vitamin C

Although many animals are able to create vitamin C within their own bodies, humans drew the short straw there and cannot perform this feat. We could say that we make this up by eating said animals, but fruits and vegetables are overwhelmingly the best providers of vitamin C. This vitamin is the most popular supplement consumed, no doubt due to collective societal flashbacks of pirate incursions and wishing for that particular fear never to return.

The more well-known association that vitamin C has is with the immune system. This is indeed part of its functionality, as well as its activity as a potent antioxidant.[25,26] It can even help restore amounts of other antioxidants like vitamin E. On the construction side, vitamin C helps with the assembly of neurotransmitters and collagen, as well as being a factor in the metabolic activity of proteins.[27,28] Furthermore, vitamin C is a valuable antihistamine with the noted benefits of supplementation and increased histamine levels due to deficiency.[29-31] Antihistamines are well known for reducing or preventing allergic reactions.

It goes without saying that we will once again mention scurvy as a potential and terrifying result of vitamin C deficiency.[32-34] After all, weakness, swollen gums, loose teeth, inadequate wound healing, joint pain, and a host of other issues are no walk in the park. Oh, and scurvy being fatal if untreated isn't so hot either.[35,36]

Where to find vitamin C: Peppers, oranges, grapefruits, kiwi, lemons, tomatoes, broccoli, cabbage, potatoes, strawberries, Brussels sprouts.

Where not to find it: 17th-century pirate ships.

Vitamin E

Vitamin E and vitamin C are often taken together. Although vitamin C dissolves in water, vitamin E dissolves in fat. Although there are many forms of vitamin E, as far as supplements go, the most appropriate way to go about taking one is a combination of gamma, alpha, beta, and delta isomers, and not as just one variant.

As many are aware, Vitamin E is a potent antioxidant.[37] Through specific enzymatic action, vitamin E can reduce the tendency of platelets to cluster together, which if done at inopportune times, can lead to a blood clot, the kind inside a blood vessel that you definitely don't want to get.[33] Vitamin E is a factor in various functions, such as metabolic processes, immune function, and the expression of genes.[38]

The primary association with a deficiency of vitamin E relates to poor neural function. Malfunctions associated with this deficiency can include a lack of coordinated voluntary movement, muscular weakness, and nerve damage.[39-46] Vitamin E deficiency is also related to a decreased red blood cell life span.[47,48] Fortunately for all involved, vitamin E deficiency is relatively rare.

Where to find vitamin E: Sunflower seeds, almonds, peanuts, hazelnuts, corn oil, olive oil.

Vitamin D

Ah yes, "Vitamin D" — an essential vitamin that should be a part of the diet, just waiting to be absorbed. We have dismissed that claim. It is certainly very important, playing roles in bone growth and restructure, preventing rickets in children, and functioning in cell growth, immune function, and reducing inflammation.[49-52] However, it shouldn't particularly be called a vitamin. The base definition of a vitamin is a nutrient, meaning something essential for the body to have that is taken in from the environment. Vitamin D is actually a secosteroid that is found in few foods naturally (but is added as a fortifying agent, when appropriate, to combat deficiency).

Vitamin D is produced in our bodies when the sun hits our skin. Therefore, although we can certainly get scant vitamin D from our foods naturally (or in large part due to the food producers putting it in), the majority of production is within the body, which somewhat takes away vitamin D's place at the vitamin table. The reason for it being called a vitamin is because the discovery happened early in the 20th century when scientists were on a roll with gaining new understandings. Vitamin D just happened to be discovered around the time other vitamins were, and so it got slapped with this wrong label. We simply added vitamin D here because it is considered part of the major vitamins, and we did not want to provide undue confusion by its absence.

Where to find vitamin D: Go outside. Barring that, fish, such as tuna and salmon, and the many dairy products that are fortified with vitamin D.

As we stated from the beginning, this is not meant to be an all-inclusive list of every action and benefit of all the nutrients that we get from food. This is simply an example of why healthy food is actually healthy. Such an endeavor would fill an encyclopedia. Further information is readily available to you, along with the relative raw scientific data. Check out reputable sources on the Internet and peruse to your heart's content until you have what it takes to be able to eat to your heart's health.

Epilogue

Thus ends our journey through a variant of medicine that is quickly growing in popularity as people find out that "Hey, this makes sense." We hope that you were both equally educated and entertained. There is a lot of information out there about the physiologic approach and its applications, and it's only necessary to put the pieces of information together in order to make an informed decision to utilize it. Remember, the information is out there for you to look through. Use the knowledge you gain to stay healthy, and most of all, make sure that you get plenty of vitamin C so that you don't turn into a pirate.

For more information, or if you have questions or comments for us, visit our website at www.dzlogic.com or call us at 1-866-225-4877.

Thanks for reading. Remember, knowledge is power. Go out and get it.

References

Part I

1. Krabbendam L, van Os J. Schizophrenia and urbanicity: a major environmental influence — conditional on genetic risk. Schizophr Bull. 2005;31:795–9.

2. Cantor-Graae E, Selten JP. Schizophrenia and migration: a meta-analysis and review. Am J Psychiatry. 2005;162:12–24.

3. Boydell J, Van Os J, McKenzie K, Allardyce J, Goel R, McCreadie RG, Murray RM. Incidence of schizophrenia in ethnic minorities in London: ecological study into interactions with environment. BMJ. 2001;323:1336.

4. Veling W, Susser E, van Os J, Mackenbach JP, Selten JP, Hoek HW. Ethnic density of neighborhoods and incidence of psychotic disorders among immigrants. Am J Psychiatry. 2008;165:66–73.

5. Moore TH, Zammit S, Lingford-Hughes A, Barnes TR, Jones PB, Burke M, Lewis G. Cannabis use and risk of psychotic or affective mental health outcomes: a systematic review. Lancet. 2007;370:319–28.

6. D'Souza DC, Abi-Saab WM, Madonick S, Forcelius-Bielen K, Doersch A, Braley G, et al. Delta-9-tetra hydrocannabinol effects in schizophrenia: implications for cognition, psychosis, and addiction. Biol Psychiatry. 2005;57:594–608.

7. Henquet C, Rosa A, Krabbendam L, Papiol S, Fananas L, Drukker M, et al. An experimental study of catechol-o-methyltransferase Val158Met moderation of delta-9-tetrahydrocannabinol-induced effects on psychosis and cognition. Neuropsychopharmacology. 2006;31:2748–57.

8. Smith CA, Harrison DJ. Association between polymorphism in gene for microsomal epoxide hydrolase and susceptibility to emphysema. Lancet. 1997;350:630–3.

9. Herder C, Roden M. Genetics of type 2 diabetes: pathophysiologic and clinical relevance. Eur J Clin Invest. 2011;41(6):679-92.

10. Kapil U. Successful efforts toward elimination iodine deficiency in India. Indian J Community Med. 2010;35(4):455-68.

Part II

1. Feldmann H, Geisbert TW. Ebola haemorrhagic fever. Lancet. 2011;377(9768):849-62.

2. Mayne L, Girod C, Weltz S. 2011 Millman Medical Index. May 2012. Available at: http://publications.milliman.com/periodicals/mmi/pdfs/milliman-medical-index-2011.pdf. Accessed April 3, 2012.

3. Starfield B. Is US health really the best in the world? JAMA. 2000;284(4):483-5.

4. Smith D. Cardiovascular disease: a historic perspective. Jpn J Vet Res. 2000;48(2-3):147-66.

5. Jacobson TA. Clinical context: current concepts of coronary heart disease management. Am J Med. 2001;110 Suppl 6A:3S-11S.

6. Held C, Iqbal R, Lear SA, Rosengren A, Islam S, Matthew J, Yusuf S. Physical activity levels, ownership of goods promoting sedentary behaviour and risk of myocardial infarction: results of the INTERHEART study. Eur Heart J. 2012 Feb;33(4):452-66.

7. Yusuf S, Hawken S, Ounpuu S, Dans T, Avezum A, Lanas F, et al. Effect of potentially modifiable risk factors associated with myocardial

infarction in 52 countries (the INTERHEART study): case-control study. Lancet. 2004 Sep 11-17;364(9438):937-52.

8. Barness LA, Opitz JM, Gilbert-Barness E. Obesity: genetic, molecular, and environmental aspects. Am J Med Genet A. 2007;143A(24):3016–34.

9. Rocchini AP. Obesity hypertension. Am J Hypertens. 2002;15(2 Pt 2):50S-2S.

10. Haslam DW, James WP. Obesity. Lancet. 2005;366(9492):1197-209.

11. Mariolis P, Rock VJ, Asman K, Merritt R, Malarcher A, Husten C, et al. Tobacco Use Among Adults --- United States, 2005. Available at: http://www.cdc.gov/mmwr/preview/mmwrhtml/mm5542a1.htm. Accessed April 3, 2012.

12. U.S. Obesity Trends. Available at: http://www.cdc.gov/obesity/data/trends.html. Accessed April 5, 2012.

13. Velazquez EJ, Lee KL, Deja MA, Jain A, Sopko G, Marchenko A, et al. Coronary-artery bypass surgery in patients with left ventricular dysfunction. N Engl J Med. 2011 Apr 28;364(17):1607–16.

14. Weintraub WS, Spertus JA, Kolm P, Maron DJ, Zhang Z, Jurkovitz C, et al. Effect of PCI on quality of life in patients with stable coronary artery disease. N Engl J Med. 2008 Aug 14;359(7):677-87.

15. Boden WE, O'Rourke RA, Teo KK, Hartigan PM, Maron DJ, Kostuk WJ, et al. Optimal medical therapy with or without PCI for stable coronary disease. N Engl J Med. 2007 Apr 12;356(15):1503-16.

16. Ornish D. Integrative Care: A Pathway to a Healthier Nation. Available at: http://www.help.senate.gov/imo/media/doc/Ornish.pdf.

17. Adams KM, Lindell KC, Kohlmeier M, Zeisel SH. Status of nutrition education in medical schools. Am J Clin Nutr. 2006;83(4):941S-4S.

18. Silver MA, Langsjoen PH, Szabo S, Patil H, Zelinger A. Statin cardiomyopathy? A potential role for Co-Enzyme Q10 therapy for statin-induced changes in diastolic LV performance: description of a clinical protocol. Biofactors. 2003;18(1-4):125-7.

19. Sauret JM, Marinides G, Wang GK. Rhabdomyolysis. Am Fam Physician. 2002;65(5):907–12.

20. Zeitlinger M, Müller M. [Clinico-pharmacologic explanation models of cerivastatin associated rhabdomyolysis]. Wien Med Wochenschr. 2003;153(11–12):250–4.

21. Muldoon MF, Ryan CM, Flory JD, Manuck SB. Effects of simvastatin on cognitive functioning. Presented at the American Heart Association Scientific Sessions. Chicago, IL, USA. 2002, Nov. 17-20.

22. Wagstaff LR, Mitton MW, Arvik BM, Doraiswamy PM. Statin-associated memory loss: analysis of 60 case reports and review of the literature. Pharmacotherapy. 2003 Jul;23(7):871-80.

23. King DS, Wilburn AJ, Wofford MR, Harrell TK, Lindley BJ, Jones DW. Cognitive impairment associated with atorvastatin and simvastatin. Pharmacotherapy. 2003 Dec;23(12):1663-7.

24. Orsi A, Sherman O, Woldeselassie Z. Simvastatin-associated memory loss. Pharmacotherapy. 2001 Jun;21(6):767-9.

25. Gaist D, García Rodríguez LA, Huerta C, Hallas J, Sindrup SH. Are users of lipid-lowering drugs at increased risk of peripheral neuropathy? Eur J Clin Pharmacol. 2001 Mar;56(12):931-3.

26. Ahmad A, Fletcher MT, Roy TM. Simvastatin-induced lupus-like syndrome. Tenn Med. 2000 Jan;93(1):21-2.

27. McPherson R, Hanna K, Agro A, Braeken A; Canadian Cerivastatin Study Group. Cerivastatin versus branded pravastatin in the treatment of primary hypercholesterolemia in primary care practice in Canada: a one-year, open-label, randomized, comparative study of efficacy, safety, and cost-effectiveness. Clin Ther. 2001 Sep;23(9):1492-507.

28. Smith GD, Song F, Sheldon TA. Cholesterol lowering and mortality: the importance of considering initial level of risk. BMJ. 1993 May 22;306(6889):1367-73.

29. Childs M, Girardot G. Evaluation of acquired data on long-term risk of hypolipidemic treatments. Arch Mal Coeur Vaiss. 1992 Sep;85 Spec No 2:129-33.

30. Banga JD. Myotoxicity and rhabdomyolisis due to statins. Ned Tijdschr Geneeskd. 2001;145(49):2371-6.

31. Simons LA, Levis G, Simons J. Apparent discontinuation rates in patients prescribed lipid-lowering drugs. Med J Aust. 1996 Feb 19;164(4):208-11.

32. Zhang D, Sun Y, Yue Z, Li Q, Meng J, Liu J, et al. Apple polysaccharides induce apoptosis in colorectal cancer cells. Int J Mol Med. 2012 Jul;30(1):100-6.

33. Available at: http://news.harvard.edu/gazette/story/2009/09/new-study-finds-45000-deaths-annually-linked-to-lack-of-health-coverage/. Accessed April 6, 2012.

Part III

1. Guerin JC. Emerging area of aging research: long-lived animals with "negligible senescence". Ann N Y Acad Sci. 2004 Jun;1019:518-20.

2. Salimpoor VN, Benovoy M, Larcher K, Dagher A, Zatorre RJ. Anatomically distinct dopamine release during anticipation and experience of peak emotion to music. Nat Neurosci. 2011; 14(2):257-62.

3. Hof PR, Mobbs CV. Handbook of the neuroscience of aging. London: Elsevier. 2009. ISBN 9780123748980.

4. Paul SM, Purdy RH. Neuroactive steroids. FASEB J. 1992 Mar;6(6):2311-22.

5. Azevedo F, Carvalho L, Grinberg L, Farfel J, Ferretti R, Leite, R, et al. Equal numbers of neuronal and nonneuronal cells make the human brain an isometrically scaled-up primate brain. J Comp Neurol. 2009 Apr 10;513(5):532-41.

6. Roberts E, Fitten LJ. Serum steroid levels in two old men with Alzheimer's disease (AD) before and after oral administration of dehydroepiandrosterone (DHEA). Pregnenolone synthesis may be ratelimiting in aging. In: Kalimi M, Regelson W, editors. The Biological Role of Dehydroepiandrosterone (DHEA). Berlin , de Gruyter, 1990;43-63.

7. Semeniuk T, Jhangri GS, Le Mellédo JM. Neuroactive steroid levels in patients with generalized anxiety disorder. J Neuropsychiatry Clin Neurosci. 2001 Summer;13(3):396-8.

8. Ballenger, JC; Davidson, JR, Lecrubier, Y, Nutt, DJ, Borkovec, TD, Rickels, K, et al. Consensus statement on generalized anxiety disorder from the International Consensus Group on Depression and Anxiety. J Clin Psychiatry. 2001;62 Suppl 11:53-8.

9. George MS, Guidotti A, Rubinow D, Pan B, Mikalauskas K, Post RM. CSF neuroactive steroids in affective disorders: pregnenolone, progesterone, and DBI. Biol Psychiatry. 1994 May 15;35(10):775-80.

10. Osuji IJ, Vera-Bolaños E, Carmody TJ, Brown ES. Pregnenolone for cognition and mood in dual diagnosis patients. Psychiatry Res. 2010 Jul 30;178(2):309-12.

11. Roberts E. Pregneolone—from Selye to Alzheimer and a model of the pregnenolone sulfate binding site on the GABAA receptor. Biochem Pharmacol. 1995 Jan 6;49(1):1-16.

12. Copeland JL, Consitt LA, Tremblay MS. Hormonal responses to endurance and resistance exercise in females aged 19-69 years. J Gerontol A Biol Sci Med Sci. 2002 Apr;57(4):B158-65.

13. Ganong WF. Review of Medical Physiology. 22nd Ed, McGraw Hill. 2005; 362.

14. The Merck Index, 13th Edition, 7798.

15. Schulman RA, Dean Carolyn. DHEA (Dehydroepiandrosterone) is a common hormone produced in the adrenal glands, the gonads, and the brain. In: Solve it with supplements. New York City: Rodale, Inc. 2007;100. ISBN 978-1-57954-942-8.

16. Dharia S, Parker CR Jr. Adrenal androgens and aging. Semin Reprod Med. 2004 Nov;22(4):361-8.

17. Bélanger A, Candas B, Dupont A, Cusan L, Diamond P, Gomez JL, et al. Changes in serum concentrations of conjugated and unconjugated steroids in 40- to 80-year-old men. J Clin Endocrinol Metab. 1994 Oct;79(4):1086-90.

18. Labrie F, Bélanger A, Cusan L, Gomez JL, Candas B. Marked decline in serum concentrations of adrenal C19 sex steroid precursors and conjugated androgen metabolites during aging. J Clin Endocrinol Metab. 1997 Aug;82(8):2396-402.

19. Barad D, Brill H, Gleicher N. Update on the use of dehydroepiandrosterone supplementation among women with diminished ovarian function. J Assist Reprod Genet. 2007 Dec;24(12):629-34.

20. Casson PR, Lindsay MS, Pisarska MD, Carson SA, Buster JE. Dehydroepiandrosterone supplementation augments ovarian stimulation in poor responders: a case series. Hum Reprod. 2000;15:2129-32.

21. Barrett-Connor E, Khaw KT Yen SS. A prospective study of dehydroepiandrosterone sulfate, mortality, and cardiovascular disease. N Eng J Med. 1986 Dec;315:1519-24.

22. Alhaj HA, Massey AE, McAllister-Williams RH. Effects of DHEA administration on episodic memory, cortisol and mood in healthy young men: a double-blind, placebo-controlled study. Psychopharmacology (Berl). 2006 Nov;188(4):541-51.

23. Bloch M, Schmidt PJ, Danaceau MA, Adams LF, Rubinow DR. Dehydroepiandrosterone treatment of midlife dysthymia. Biol Psychiatry. 1999 Jun 15;45(12):1533-41.

24. Wolkowitz OM, Reus VI, Roberts E, Manfredi F, Chan T, Raum WJ, et al. Dehydroepiandrosterone (DHEA) treatment of depression. Biol Psychiatry. 1997 Feb 1;41(3):311-8.

25. Salom MG, Jabaloyas JM. [Testosterone deficit syndrome and erectile dysfunction]. Arch Esp Urol. 2010 Oct;63(8):663-70.

26. Panay N, Al-Azzawi F, Bouchard C, Davis SR, Eden J, Lodhi I, et al. Testosterone treatment of HSDD in naturally menopausal women: the ADORE study. Climacteric. 2010 Apr;13(2):121-31.

27. Malkin CJ, Pugh PJ, Morris PD, Asif S, Jones TH, Channer KS. Low serum testosterone and increased mortality in men with coronary heart disease. Heart. 2010 Nov;96(22):1821-5.

28. Iellamo F, Volterrani M, Caminiti G, Karam R, Massaro R, Fini M, et al. Testosterone therapy in women with chronic heart failure: a pilot double-blind, randomized, placebo-controlled study. J Am Coll Cardiol. 2010 Oct 12;56(16):1310-6.

29. Białek M, Zaremba P, Borowicz KK, Czuczwar SJ. Neuroprotective role of testosterone in the nervous system. Pol J Pharmacol. 2004 Sep-Oct;56(5):509-18.

30. Pentikäinen V, Erkkilä K, Suomalainen L, Parvinen M, Dunkel L. Estradiol acts as a germ cell survival factor in the human testis in vitro. J Clin Endocrinol Metab. 2000 May;85(5):2057-67.

31. Craig MC, Murphy DG. Estrogen therapy and Alzheimer's dementia. Ann N Y Acad Sci. 2010 Sep;1205:245-53.

32. Douma SL, Husband C, O'Donnell ME, Barwin BN, Woodend AK. Estrogen-related mood disorders: reproductive life cycle factors. ANS Adv Nurs Sci. 2005 Oct-Dec;28(4):364-75.

33. Sánchez MG, Bourque M, Morissette M, Di Paolo T. Steroids-dopamine interactions in the pathophysiology and treatment of CNS disorders. CNS Neurosci Ther. 2010 Jun;16(3):e43-71.

34. Hu Z, Li Y, Fang M, Wai MS, Yew DT. Exogenous progesterone: a potential therapeutic candidate in CNS injury and neurodegeneration. Curr Med Chem. 2009;16(11):1418-25.

35. Oettel M, Mukhopadhyay AK. Progesterone: the forgotten hormone in men? Aging Male. 2004 Sep;7(3):236-57.

Part IV

1. Fournier A, Berrino F, Clavel-Chapelon F. Unequal risks for breast cancer associated with different hormone replacement therapies: results from the E3N cohort study. Breast Cancer Res Treat. 2008 Jan;107(1):103-11.

2. Rossouw JE, Anderson GL, Prentice RL, LaCroix AZ, Kooperberg C, Stefanick ML, et al. Risks and benefits of estrogen plus progestin in healthy postmenopausal women: principal results From the Women's Health Initiative randomized controlled trial. JAMA. 2002 Jul 17;288(3):321-33.

3. Ziel HK, Finkle WD. Increased risk of endometrial carcinoma among users of conjugated estrogens. N Engl J Med. 1975 Dec 4;293(23):1167-70.

4. Garcia-Santos G, Martin V, Rodriguez-Blanco J, Herrera F, Casado-Zapico S, Sanchez-Sanchez AM, et al. Fas/Fas ligand regulation mediates cell death in human Ewing's sarcoma cells treated with melatonin. Br J Cancer. 2012;106(7):1288-96.

5. Available at: http://www.nlm.nih.gov/medlineplus/ency/article/002423.htm. Accessed April 12, 2012.

6. Rude RK, Shils ME. Magnesium. In: Shils ME, Shike M, Ross AC, Caballero B, Cousins RJ, eds. Modern Nutrition in Health and Disease. 10th ed. Baltimore: Lippincott Williams & Wilkins. 2006;223-247.

7. Blaylock RL. Health and Nutrition Secrets. Health Pres. 2006;395. ISBN 978-0-929173-48-1.

8. Available   at: http://www.ars.usda.gov/Services/docs.htm?docid=15677. Accessed April 12, 2012.

9. Available at: http://ehealthmd.com/content/what-causes-prostate-enlarge. Accessed April 13, 2012.

10. Berdanier CD, Dwyer JT, Feldman EB. Handbook of Nutrition and Food. Boca Raton, Florida: CRC Press. 2007. ISBN 0-8493-9218-7.

11. Age-Related Eye Disease Study Research Group. A randomized, placebo-controlled, clinical trial of high-dose supplementation with vitamins C and E, beta carotene, and zinc for age-related macular degeneration and vision loss: AREDS report no. 8. Arch Ophthalmol. 2001 Oct;119(10):1417-36.

Part V

1. Available at: http://www.sigmaaldrich.com/Area_of_Interest/Biochemicals/Enzyme_Explorer/Key_Resources/Plasma__Blood_Protein/Lipoprotein_Function.html Accessed April 29, 2012.

2. Martin U, Davies C, Hayavi S, Hartland A, Dunne F. Is normal pregnancy atherogenic? Clin Sci (Lond). 1999 Apr;96(4):421-5.

3. Warth MR, Arky RA, Knopp RH. Lipid metabolism in pregnancy. II. Altered lipid composition in intermediage, very low, low and high-density lipoprotein fractions. J Clin Endocrinol Metab. 1975 Oct;41(4):649-55.

4. Sitadevi C, Patrudu MB, Kumar YM, Raju GR, Suryaprabha K. Longitudinal study of serum lipids and lipoproteins in normal pregnancy and puerperium. Trop Geogr Med. 1981 Sep;33(3):219-23.

5. Brizzi P, Tonolo G, Esposito F, Puddu L, Dessole S, Maioli M, et al. Lipoprotein metabolism during normal pregnancy. Am J Obstet Gynecol. 1999 Aug;181(2):430-4.

6. Troisi A, Moles A, Panepuccia L, Lo Russo D, Palla G, Scucchi S. Serum cholesterol levels and mood symptoms in the postpartum period. Psychiatry Res. 2002 Apr 15;109(3):213-9.

7. Mizuno O, Yokoyama T, Tsutsumi N. The changes of serum total cholesterol, HDL-cholesterol and atherogenic index in postpartum. Nippon Sanka Fujinka Gakkai Zasshi. 1984 Dec;36(12):2593-7.

8. Erkkola R, Viikari J, Irjala K, Solakivi-Jaakkola T. One-year follow-up of lipoprotein metabolism after pregnancy. Biol Res Pregnancy Perinatol. 1986;7(2):47-51.

9. Smolarczyk R, Romejko E, Wójcicka-Jagodzińska J, Czajkowski K, Teliga-Czajkowska J, Piekarski P. Lipid metabolism in women with threatened abortion. Ginekol Pol. 1996 Oct;67(10):481-7.

10. Samánek M, Urbanová Z. Cholesterol and triglyceride levels and their development from 2 to 17 years of age. Cas Lek Cesk. 1997 Jun 12;136(12):380-5.

11. Rodkiewicz B, Szotowa W, Woynarowska B, Cerańska-Goszczyńska H, Ignar-Golinowska B, Pułtorak M.. Serum cholesterol levels in children aged 4-14 years. Probl Med Wieku Rozwoj. 1984;13:95-102.

12. Lin CC, Lai MM, Liu CS, Li TC. Serum cholesterol levels and prevalence of hypercholesterolemia in school-aged Taiwanese children and adolescents: the Taichung Study. Zhonghua Yi Xue Za Zhi (Taipei). 1999 Nov;62(11):787-94.

13. Lerman-Garber I, Sepúlveda-Amor JA, Tapia-Conyer R, Magos-López C, Cardoso-Saldaña G, Zamora-González J, et al. Cholesterol levels and prevalence of hypercholesterolemia in Mexican children and teenagers. Atherosclerosis. 1993 Nov;103(2):195-203.

14. Suthutvoravut   U, Charoenkiatkul   S, Chitchumroonchokchai C, Kosulwat V, Mahachoklertwattana P, Rojroongwasinkul N. Elevated serum cholesterol levels in Bangkok children and adolescents. J Med Assoc Thai. 1999 Nov;82 Suppl 1:S117-21.

15. Lehtonen A, Viikari J. Serum lipids in soccer and ice-hockey players. Metabolism. 1980 Jan;29(1):36-9.

16. Boston PF, Dursun SM, Reveley MA. Cholesterol and mental disorder. Br J Psychiatry. 1996 Dec;169(6):682-9.

17. Bostom AG, Cupples LA, Jenner JL, Ordovas JM, Seman LJ, Wilson PW, et al. Lipoprotein(a)-cholesterol and coronary heart disease in the Framingham Heart Study. Clin Chem. 1999;45(7):1039-46.

18. Papassotiropoulos A, Hawellek B, Frahnert C, Rao GS, Rao ML. The risk of acute suicidality in psychiatric inpatients increases with low plasma cholesterol. Pharmacopsychiatry. 1999;32(1):1-4.

19. Gould AL, Rossouw JE, Santanello NC, Heyse JF, Furberg CD. Cholesterol reduction yields clinical benefit. A new look at old data. Circulation. 1995;91(8):2274-82.

20. Jakovljević M, Reiner Z, Milicić D. Mental disorders, treatment response, mortality and serum cholesterol: a new holistic look at old data. Psychiatr Danub. 2007 Dec;19(4):270-81.

21. Windler E, Ewers-Grabow U, Thiery J, Walli A, Seidel D, Greten H. The prognostic value of hypocholesterolemia in hospitalized patients. Clin Investig. 1994 Dec;72(12):939-43.

22. Onder G, Landi F, Volpato S, Fellin R, Carbonin P, Gambassi G, et al. Serum cholesterol levels and in-hospital mortality in the elderly. Am J Med. 2003 Sep;115(4):265-71.

23. Corti MC, Guralnik JM, Salive ME, Harris T, Ferrucci L, Glynn RJ, et al. Clarifying the direct relation between total cholesterol levels and death from coronary heart disease in older persons. Ann Intern Med. 1997 May 15;126(10):753-60.

24. Krumholz HM, Seeman TE, Merrill SS, Mendes de Leon CF, Vaccarino V, Silverman DI, et al. Lack of association between cholesterol and coronary heart disease mortality and morbidity and all-cause mortality in persons older than 70 years. JAMA. 1994 Nov 2;272(17):1335-40.

25. Stemmermann GN, Chyou PH, Kagan A, Nomura AM, Yano K. Serum cholesterol and mortality among Japanese-American men. The Honolulu (Hawaii) Heart Program. Arch Intern Med. 1991 May;151(5):969-72.

26. Navab M, Van Lenten BJ, Reddy ST, Fogelman AM. High-density lipoprotein and the dynamics of atherosclerotic lesions. Circulation. 2001 Nov 13;104(20):2386-7.

27. Siemianowicz K, Gminski J, Stajszczyk M, Wojakowski W, Goss M, Machalski M, et al. Serum total cholesterol and triglycerides levels in patients with lung cancer. Int J Mol Med. 2000 Feb;5(2):201-5.

28. Williams RR, Sorlie PD, Feinleib M, McNamara PM, Kannel WB, Dawber TR. Cancer incidence by levels of cholesterol. JAMA. 1981 Jan 16;245(3):247-52.

29. Törnberg SA, Carstensen JM, Holm LE. Risk of stomach cancer in association with serum cholesterol and beta-lipoprotein. Acta Oncol. 1988;27(1):39-42.

30. Knekt P, Reunanen A, Aromaa A, Heliövaara M, Hakulinen T, Hakama M. Serum cholesterol and risk of cancer in a cohort of 39,000 men and women. Clin Epidemiol. 1988;41(6):519-30.

31. Goldstein MR, Mascitelli L. Do statins decrease cardiovascular disease at the expense of increasing cancer? Int J Cardiol. 2009 Apr 3;133(2):254-5.

32. Iribarren C, Jacobs DR Jr, Sidney S, Claxton AJ, Gross MD, Sadler M, et al. Serum total cholesterol and risk of hospitalization, and death from respiratory disease. Int J Epidemiol. 1997 Dec;26(6):1191-202.

33. Fraunberger P, Schaefer S, Werdan K, Walli AK, Seidel D. Reduction of circulating cholesterol and apolipoprotein levels during sepsis. Clin Chem Lab Med. 1999 Mar;37(3):357-62.

34. Claxton AJ, Jacobs DR Jr, Iribarren C, Welles SL, Sidney S, Feingold KR. Association between serum total cholesterol and HIV infection in a high-risk cohort of young men. J Acquir Immune Defic Syndr Hum Retrovirol. 1998 Jan 1;17(1):51-7.

35. Shor-Posner G, Basit A, Lu Y, Cabrejos C, Chang J, Fletcher M, et al. Hypocholesterolemia is associated with immune dysfunction in early human immunodeficiency virus-1 infection. Am J Med. 1993 May;94(5):515-9.

36. Leardi S, Altilia F, Delmonaco S, Cianca G, Pietroletti R, Simi M. Blood levels of cholesterol and postoperative septic complications. Ann Ital Chir. 2000 Mar-Apr;71(2):233-7.

37. Ormiston T, Wolkowitz OM, Reus VI, Johnson R, Manfredi F. Hormonal changes with cholesterol reduction: a double-blind pilot study. J Clin Pharm Ther. 2004 Feb;29(1):71-3.

38. Dzugan SA, Rozakis GW, Dzugan SS, Smith RA. Hormonorestorative therapy is a promising method for hypercholesterolemia treatment. Approaches to Aging Control. 2009;13:12-9.

39. Dzugan SA, Rozakis GW, Dzugan KS, Emhof L, Dzugan SS, Xydas C, et al. Correction of Steroidopenia as a New Method of Hypercholesterolemia Treatment. Neuroendocrinol Lett (NEL). 2011;32(1):77-81.

40. Smith D. Cardiovascular disease: a historic perspective. Jpn J Vet Res. 2000 Nov;48(2-3):147-66.

41. Jacobson TA. Clinical context: current concepts of coronary heart disease management. Am J Med. 2001 Apr 16;110 Suppl 6A:3S-11S.

42. Weiner SD, Reis ED, Kerstein MD. Peripheral arterial disease. Medical management in primary care practice. Geriartrics. 2001 Apr;56(4):20-2, 25-6, 29-30.

43. Soska V. Pharmacotherapy of hyperlipoproteinemia. Vnitr Lek. 2000 Sep;46(9):565-8.

44. Hanefeld M, Hora C, Schulze J, Rothe G, Barthel U, Haller H. Reduced incidence of cardiovascular complications and mortality in hyperlipoproteinemia (HLP) with effective lipid correction. The Dresden HLP study. Atherosclerosis. 1984 Oct;53(1):47-58.

45. Vogel RA, Corretti MC, Gellman J. Cholesterol, cholesterol lowering, and endothelial function. Prog Cardiovasc Dis. 1998 Sep-Oct;41(2):117-36

46. Lopez-Sendon JL, Rubio R, Lopez de Sa E, Delcan JL. Why the cardiologists should be interested in lipids? Rev Esp Cardiol. 1995;48 Suppl 2:23-32.

47. Hughes K. Screening for and treatment of hypercholesterolemia – a review. Ann Acad Med Singapore. 1997 Mar;26(2):215-20.

48. Yang YH, Kao SM, Chan KW. A retrospective drug utilization of antihyperlipidaemic agents in a medical center in Taiwan. J Clin Pharm Ther. 1997 Aug;22(4):291-9.

49. Turpin G, Bruckert E. Management of atherogenic hyperlipidemia. Ann Cardiol Angeiol (Paris). 1998 Nov;47(9):627-32.

50. Bancarz A, Jolda-Mydlovska B, Swidnicka-Szuszkowska B. [Pharmacological treatment of lipid disorders according to present clinical studies]. Pol Merkur Lekarski. 1998 Sep;5(27):162-6.

51. Bachmann GA. Androgen cotherapy in menopause: evolving benefits and challenges. Am J Obstet Gynecol. 1999 Mar;180(3 Pt 2):S308-11.

52. Ciepluch R, Czestochowska E. Hormonal replacement therapy and body weight in postmenopausal women. Pol Merkur Lekarski. 1997 Jan;2(9):188-90.

53. Regelson W, Loria R, Kalimi M. Hormonal intervention: "buffer hormones" or "state dependency". The role of dehydroepiandrosterone (DHEA), thyroid hormone, estrogen and hypophysectomy in aging. Ann NY Acad Sci. 1988;521:260-73.

54. Morales AJ, Nolan JJ, Nelson JC, Yen SS. Effects of replacement dose of dehydroepiandrosterone in men and women of advancing age. J Clin Endocrinol Metab. 1994. Jun;78(6):1360-7.

55. Takahashi K, Manabe A, Okada M, Kurioka H, Kanasaki H, Miyazaki K. Efficacy and safety of oral estriol for managing postmenopausal symptoms. Maturitas. 2000 Feb 15;34(2):169-77.

56. Haddock BL, Marshak HP, Mason JJ, Blix G. The effect of hormone replacement therapy and exercise on cardiovascular disease risk factors in postmenopausal women. Sports Med. 2000. Jan;29(1):39-49.

57. Kummerow FA, Olinescu RM, Fleischer L, Handler B, Shinkareva SV. The relationship of oxidized lipids to coronary artery stenosis. Atherosclerosis. 2000;149:181-190.

58. Bratus' VV, Talaieva TV, Lomakovs'kyĭ OM, Tretiak IV, Radalovs'ka NV. Modified lipoproteins – their types and role in atherogenesis. Fiziol Zh. 2000;46:73-81.

59. Haug A, Hostmark AT, Spydevold O. Plasma lipoprotein responses to castration and androgen substitution in rats. Metabolism. 1984;33:465-470.

60. Hänggi W, Birkhäuser MH, Malek A, Peheim E, von Hospenthal JU. Cyclical gestagen (MPA) supplement for continuous transdermal or oral estrogen substitution in postmenopause: modification of serum lipids. Geburtshilfe Frauenheilkd. 1993;53:709-14.

61. Dzugan SA, Smith RA. Broad spectrum restoration in natural steroid hormones as possible treatment for hypercholesterolemia. Bull Urg Rec Med. 2002;3: 278-84.

62. Dzugan SA, Smith RA. Hypercholesterolemia treatment: a new hypothesis or just an accident? Med Hypotheses. 2002;59:751-6.

63. Dzugan SA. Hypercholesterolemia treatment: a new hypothesis or just an accident. In: Anti-Aging Therapeutics. Vol. 6. Chicago, IL, USA. 2004;89-98.

64. Dzugan SA, Smith RA, Kuznetsov AS. A new statin free method of hypercholesterolemia. Health Donbass. 2004;4:19-25.

65. Dzugan SA. Hypercholesterolemia Treatment: a New Statin Free Method. In: Anti-Aging Therapeutics. Vol. 9. Chicago, IL, USA. 2007;117-25.

66. Dzugan SA, Rozakis GW, Dzugan SS, Smith RA. Hormonorestorative therapy is a promising method for hypercholesterolemia treatment. Approaches to Aging Control. 2009;13:12-9.

Part VI

1. Krippendorf, BB; Riley, DA. Distinguishing unloading-versus reloading-induced changes in rat soleus muscle. Muscle Nerve. 1993;16(1):99–108.

2. St Pierre BA, Tidball JG. Differential response of macrophage subpopulations to soleus muscle reloading following rat hindlimb suspension. J Appl Physiol. 1994 Jul;77(1):290-7.

3. Tidball JG, Berchenko E, Frenette J. Macrophage invasion does not contribute to muscle membrane injury during inflammation. J Leukoc Biol. 1999 Apr;65(4):492-8.

4. Brechot N, Gomez E, Bignon M, Khallou-Laschet J, Dussiot M, Cazes A, et al. Modulation of Macrophage Activation State Protects Tissue from Necrosis during Critical Limb Ischemia in Thrombospondin-1-Deficient Mice. PLoS One. 2008;3(12):e3950.

5. Committee to Review Dietary Reference Intakes for Vitamin D and Calcium, Food and Nutrition Board, Institute of Medicine. Dietary Reference Intakes for Calcium and Vitamin D. Washington, DC: National Academy Press. 2010.

6. Kudenchuk PJ, Maynard C, Martin JS, Wirkus M, Weaver WD. Comparison of presentation, treatment, and outcome of acute myocardial infarction in men versus women (the Myocardial Infarction Triage and Intervention Registry). Am J Cardiol. 1996;78:9–14.

7. Charney P, ed. Coronary artery disease in women: what all physicians need to know. Philadelphia: American College of Physicians. 1999.

8. Lesser M. Testosterone propionate therapy in one hundred cases of angina pectoris. J Clin Endocrinol. 1946;6:549-57.

9. Wu SZ, Weng XZ. Therapeutic effects of an androgenic preparation on myocardial ischemia and cardiac function in 62 elderly male coronary heart disease patients. Chin Med J (Engl). 1993;106:415-8.

10. Phillips GB, Pinkernell BH, Jing TY. The association of hypotestosteronemia with coronary artery disease in men. Arterioscler Thromb. 1994;14:701-6.

11. Winkler U. Effects of androgens on haemostasis. Maturitas. 1996;24:147-55.

12. Iellamo F, Volterrani M, Caminiti G, Karam R, Massaro R, Fini M, et al. Testosterone therapy in women with chronic heart failure: a pilot double-blind, randomized, placebo-controlled study. J Am Coll Cardiol. 2010 Oct 12;56(16):1310-6.

13. Stephens N, Parsons A, Schofield P, Kelly F, Cheeseman K, Mitchinson MJ. Randomised controlled trial of vitamin E in patients with coronary disease: Cambridge Heart Antioxidant Study (CHAOS). The Lancet. 1996;347:781-6.

14. Axford-Gately R, Wilson G. Myocardial infarct size reduction by single high doses or repeated low dose vitamin E supplementation in rabbits. Can J Cardiol. 1993;9:94-8.

15. DeMaio S, King Sd, Lembo N, Roubin GS, Hearn JA, Bhagavan HN, et al. Vitamin E supplementation, plasma lipids and incidence of restenosis after percutaneous transluminal coronary angioplasty (PCTA). J Am Coll Nutr. 1992;11:68-73.

16. Rapola J, Virtamo J, Haukka J, Heinonen OP, Albanes D, Taylor PR, et al. Effect of vitamin E and beta carotene on the incidence of angina pectoris. JAMA. 1996;275:693-8.

17. Steiner M. Influence of vitamin E on platelet function in humans. J Am Coll Nutr. 1991;10:466-73.

18. Enstrom JE, Kanim LE, Klein MA. Vitamin C intake and mortality among a sample of the United States population. Epidemiology. 1992;3:194-202.

19. McCully K. The Homocysteine Revolution. Keats Publishing, Inc. 1997.

20. McCully K. Homocysteine, folate, vitamin B6, and cardiovascular disease (editorial). JAMA. 1998;279:392-3.

21. Verhoef P, Hennekens CH, Malinow MR, Kok FJ, Willett WC, Stampfer MJ. A prospective study of plasma homocyst(e)ine and risk of myocardial infarction in US physicians. JAMA. 1992;268:877-81.

22. Stampfer M, Malinow M. Can lowering homocysteine levels reduce cardiovascular risk? N Engl J Med. 1995;332:328-9.

23. Bélanger A, Candas B, Dupont A, Cusan L, Diamond P, Gomez JL, et al. Changes in serum concentrations of conjugated and unconjugated steroids in 40- to 80-year-old men. J Clin Endocrinol Metab. 1994 Oct;79(4):1086-90.

24. Labrie F, Bélanger A, Cusan L, Gomez JL, Candas B. Marked decline in serum concentrations of adrenal C19 sex steroid precursors and conjugated androgen metabolites during aging. J Clin Endocrinol Metab. 1997 Aug;82(8):2396-402.

25. Regelson W, Colman C. The Superhormone Promise. New York, Simon & Schuster. 1996.

26. Salom MG, Jabaloyas JM. [Testosterone deficit syndrome and erectile dysfunction]. Arch Esp Urol. 2010 Oct;63(8):663-70.

27. Nikoobakht M, Pourkasmaee M, Nasseh H. The relationship between lipid profile and erectile dysfunction. Urol J. 2005 Winter;2(1):40-4.

28. Vrentzos GE, Paraskevas KI, Mikhailidis DP. Dyslipidemia as a risk factor for erectile dysfunction. Curr Med Chem. 2007;14(16):1765-70.

29. Padrón RS, Más J, Zamora R, Riverol F, Licea M, Mallea L, et al. Lipids and testicular function. Int Urol Nephrol. 1989;21(5):515-9.

30. Rizvi K, Hampson JP, Harvey JN. Do lipid-lowering drugs cause erectile dysfunction? A systematic review. Fam Pract. 2002 Feb;19(1):95-8.

31. Carvajal A, Macias D, Sáinz M, Ortega S, Martín Arias LH, Velasco A, et al. HMG CoA reductase inhibitors and impotence: two case series from the Spanish and French drug monitoring systems. Drug Saf. 2006;29(2):143-9.

32. Morgentaler A, Bruning CO 3rd, DeWolf WC. Occult prostate cancer in men with low serum testosterone levels. JAMA. 1996 Dec 18;276(23):1904-6.

33. Schatzl G, Madersbacher S, Haitel A, Gsur A, Preyer M, Haidinger G, et al. Associations of serum testosterone with microvessel density, androgen receptor density and androgen receptor gene polymorphism in prostate cancer. J Urol. 2003 Apr;169(4):1312-5.

34. Vatten LJ, Ursin G, Ross RK, Stanczyk FZ, Lobo RA, Harvei S, et al. Androgens in serum and the risk of prostate cancer: a nested case-control study from the Janus serum bank in Norway. Cancer Epidemiol Biomarkers Prev. 1997 Nov;6(11):967-9.

35. Chodak GW, Vogelzang NJ, Caplan RJ, Soloway M, Smith JA. Independent prognostic factors in patients with metastatic (stage D2) prostate cancer. The Zoladex Study Group. JAMA. 1991 Feb 6;265(5):618-21.

36. MacGregor, EA. Prevention and treatment of menstrual migraine. Drugs. 2010;70(14):1799–818.

37. Lay CL, Broner SW. Migraine in women. Neurol Clin. 2009 May;27(2):503-11.

38. Stovner LJ, Zwart JA, Hagen K, Terwindt GM, Pascual J. Epidemiology of headache in Europe. Eur J Neurol. 2006 Apr;13(4):333-45.

39. Bartels EM, Dreyer L, Jacobsen S, Jespersen A, Bliddal H, Danneskiold-Samsøe B. [Fibromyalgia, diagnosis and prevalence. Are gender differences explainable?]. Ugeskr Laeger. 2009;171(49):3588–92.

40. Olin R. Fibromyalgia. A neuro-immuno-endocrinologic syndrome? Lakartidningen. 1995 Feb 22;92(8):755-8.

41. Schochat T, Beckmann C. Sociodemographic characteristics, risk factors and reproductive history in subjects with fibromyalgia—results of a population-based case-control study. Z Rheumatol. 2003;62(1):46-59.

42. Adler GK, Manfredsdottir VF, Creskoff KW. Neuroendocrine abnormalities in fibromyalgia. Curr Pain Headache Rep. 2002 Aug;6(4):289-98.

43. Hudson JI, Goldenberg DL, Pope HG Jr, Keck PE Jr, Schlesinger L. Comorbidity of fibromyalgia with medical and psychiatric disorders. Am J Med. 1992 Apr;92(4):363-7.

44. Matsumoto Y. Fibromyalgia syndrome. Nippon Rinsho. 1999 Feb;57(2):364-9.

45. Russo EB. Clinical endocannabinoid deficiency (CECD): can this concept explain therapeutic benefits of cannabis in migraine, fibromyalgia, irritable bowel syndrome and other treatment-resistant conditions? Neuro Endocrinol Lett. 2004 Feb-Apr;25(1-2):31-9.

46. Nicolodi M, Sicuteri F. Fibromyalgia and migraine, two faces of the same mechanism. Serotonin as the common clue for pathogenesis and therapy. Adv Exp Med Biol. 1996;398:373-9.

47. Thompson D, Lettich L, Takeshita J. Fibromyalgia: an overview. Curr Psychiatry Rep. 2003 Jul;5(3):211-7.

48. Pongratz D, Spath M. Fibromyalgia. Fortschr Neurol Psychiatr. 2001 Apr;69(4):189-93.

49. Hug C, Gerber NJ. Fibromyalgia syndrome, a frequently misdiagnosed entity. Schweiz Med Wochenschr. 1990 Mar 24;120(12):395-401.

50. Moldofsky H. Management of sleep disorders in fibromyalgia. Rheum Dis Clin North Am. 2002 May;28(2):353-65.

51. Rohr UD, Herold J. Melatonin deficiencies in women. Maturitas. 2002 Apr 15;41 Suppl 1:S85-104.

52. Available at: http://arthritis.about.com/od/rheumatoidarthritis/a/rheumatoidlun g.htm. Accessed April 22, 2012.

53. de Groot K. [Renal manifestations in rheumatic diseases]. Internist (Berl). 2007;48(8):779–85.

54. Wolfe F, Mitchell DM, Sibley JT, Fries JF, Bloch DA, Williams CA, et al. The mortality of rheumatoid arthritis. Arthritis Rheum. 1994 Apr;37(4):481-94.

55. Aviña-Zubieta JA, Choi HK, Sadatsafavi M, Etminan M, Esdaile JM, Lacaille D. "Risk of cardiovascular mortality in patients with rheumatoid arthritis: a meta-analysis of observational studies". Arthritis Rheum. 2008 Dec 15;59(12):1690-7.

56. Baecklund E, Iliadou A, Askling J, Ekbom A, Backlin C, Granath F, et al. Association of chronic inflammation, not its treatment, with increased lymphoma risk in rheumatoid arthritis. Arthritis Rheum. 2006 Mar;54(3):692-701.

57. Franklin J, Lunt M, Bunn D, Symmons D, Silman, A. Incidence of lymphoma in a large primary care derived cohort of cases of inflammatory polyarthritis. Ann Rheum Dis. 2006 May;65(5):617-22.

58. Available at: http://www.nice.org.uk/nicemedia/pdf/CG059FullGuideline.pdf. Accessed April 22, 2012.

59. Centers for Disease Control and Prevention (CDC) (February 2001). Prevalence of disabilities and associated health conditions among adults—United States, 1999. MMWR Morb Mortal Wkly Rep. 50(7):120–5.

60. Kolf CM, Cho E, Tuan RS. Mesenchymal stromal cells. Biology of adult mesenchymal stem cells: regulation of niche, selfrenewal and differentiation. Arthritis Res Ther. 2007;9:204.

61. Phinney DG, Prockop DJ. Concise review: mesenchymal stem/ multipotent stromal cells: the state of transdifferentiation and modes of tissue repair—current views. Stem Cells. 2007;25:2896–902.

62. Satija NK, Gurudutta GU, Sharma S, Afrin F, Gupta P, Verma YK, et al. Mesenchymal stem cells: molecular targets for tissue engineering. Stem Cells Dev. 2007;16:7–23.

63. Suzuki M, Wright LS, Marwah P, Lardy HA, Svendsen CN. Mitotic and neurogenic effects of dehydroepiandrosterone (DHEA) on human neural stem cell cultures derived from the fetal cortex. Proc Natl Acad Sci U S A. 2004 Mar 2;101(9):3202-7.

64. Pinnock SB, Lazic SE, Wong HT, Wong IH, Herbert J. Synergistic effects of dehydroepiandrosterone and fluoxetine on proliferation of progenitor cells in the dentate gyrus of the adult male rat. Neuroscience. 2009 Feb 18;158(4):1644-51.

65. Han K, Lee JE, Kwon SJ, Park SY, Shim SH, Kim H, et al. Human amnion-derived mesenchymal stem cells are a potential source for uterine stem cell therapy. Cell Prolif. 2008 Oct;41(5):709-25.

66. Labombarda F, González SL, Lima A, Roig P, Guennoun R, Schumacher M, et al. Effects of progesterone on oligodendrocyte progenitors, oligodendrocyte transcription factors, and myelin proteins following spinal cord injury. Glia. 2009 Jun;57(8):884-97.

67. De Nicola AF, Gonzalez SL, Labombarda F, Deniselle MC, Garay L, Guennoun R, et al. Progesterone treatment of spinal cord injury: Effects on receptors, neurotrophins, and myelination. J Mol Neurosci. 2006;28(1):3-15.

68. Labombarda F, Gonzalez S, Gonzalez Deniselle MC, Garay L, Guennoun R, Chumacher M, et al. Progesterone increases the expression of myelin basic protein and the number of cells showing NG2 immunostaining in the lesioned spinal cord. J Neurotrauma. 2006 Feb;23(2):181-92.

69. Foresta C, Caretta N, Lana A, De Toni L, Biagioli A, Ferlin A, et al. Reduced number of circulating endothelial progenitor cells in hypogonadal men. J Clin Endocrinol Metab. 2006 Nov;91(11):4599-602.

70. Siiteri P, Wilson JD. Testosterone formation and metabolism during male sexual differentiation in the human embryo. J Clin Endocrinol Metab. 1974;38:113.

71. Golomb BA, Stattin H, Mednick S. Low cholesterol and violent crime. J Psychiatr Res. 2000 Jul-Oct;34(4-5):301-9.

72. Atmaca M, Kuloglu M, Tezcan E, Ustundag B, Bayik Y. Serum leptin and cholesterol levels in patients with bipolar disorder. Neuropsychobiology. 2002;46(4):176-9.

73. Cassidy F, Carroll BJ. Hypocholesterolemia during mixed manic episodes. Eur Arch Psychiatry Clin Neurosci. 2002 Jun;252(3):110-4.

74. Fukui M, Soh J, Tanaka M, Kitagawa Y, Hasegawa G, Yoshikawa T. Low serum testosterone concentration in middle-aged men with type 2 diabetes. Endocr J. 2007;54:871-7.

75. Grossman M, Thomas MC, Panagiotopoulos S, Sharpe K, Macisaac RJ, Clark S, et al. Low testosterone levels are common and associated with insulin resistance in men with diabetes. J Clin Endocrinol Metab. 2008;93(5):1834-40.

76. Haffner SM, Shaten J, Stern MP, Smith GD, Kuller L. Low levels of sex hormone-binding globulin and testosterone predict the development of non-insulin-dependent diabetes mellitus in men. MRFIT Research Group. Multiple Risk Factor Intervention Trial. Am J Epidemiol. 1996;143:889-97.

77. Kapoor D, Goodwin E, Channer KS, Jones TH. Testosterone replacement therapy improves insulin resistance, glycaemic control, visceral adiposity and hypercholesterolaemia in hypogonadal men with type 2 diabetes. Eur J Endocrinol. 2006;154:899-906.

78. Picard F, Wanatabe M, Schoonjans K, Lydon J, O'Malley BW, Auwerx J. Progesterone receptor knockout mice have an improved glucose homeostasis secondary to beta -cell proliferation. Proc Natl Acad Sci U S A. 2002 Nov 26;99(24):15644-8.

Part VII

1. Available at: http://www.iaso.org/iotf/obesity/. Accessed April 22, 2012.

2. Vertuani S, Angusti A, Manfredini S. The antioxidants and pro-antioxidants network: an overview. Curr Pharm Des. 2004;10(14):1677-94.

3. Futoryan T, Gilchrest BE. Retinoids and the skin. Nutr Rev. 1994;52:299-310.

4. Ross AC. Vitamin A and retinoids. In: Modern Nutrition in Health and Disease. 9th Edition (edited by Shils ME, Olson J, Shike M, Ross AC). Lippincott Williams and Wilkins, New York. 1999;305-27.

5. Ross AC, Stephensen CB. Vitamin A and retinoids in antiviral responses. FASEB J. 1996;10:979-85.

6. Semba RD. The role of vitamin A and related retinoids in immune function. Nutr Rev. 1998;56:S38-48.

7. Ross DA. Vitamin A and public health: Challenges for the next decade. Proc Nutr Soc. 1998;57:159-65.

8. Harbige LS. Nutrition and immunity with emphasis on infection and autoimmune disease. Nutr Health. 1996;10:285-312.

9. Sommer A. Nutritional Blindness: Xeropthalmia and Keratomalacia. Oxford University Press, London and New York. 1982.

10. Ross AC. Vitamin A status: Relationship to immunity and the antibody. Proc Soc Exp Biol Med. 1992;200:303-20.

11. Stephens D, Jackson PL, Gutierrez Y. Subclinical vitamin A deficiency: A potentially unrecognized problem in the United States. Pediatr Nurs. 1996;22:377-89.

12. Butler JC, Havens PL, Sowell AL, Huff DL, Peterson DE, Day SE, et al. Measles severity and serum retinol (vitamin A) concentration among children in the United States. Pediatrics. 1993;91:1176-81.

13. Herbert V. Vitamin B12 in Present Knowledge in Nutrition. 17th ed. Washington, DC: International Life Sciences Institute Press. 1996.

14. Herbert V, Das K. Vitamin B12 in Modern Nutrition in Health and Disease. 8th ed. Baltimore, MD: Williams & Wilkins. 1994.

15. Zittoun J, Zittoun R. Modern clinical testing strategies in cobalamin and folate deficiency. Sem Hematol. 1999;36:35-46.

16. Combs G. Vitamin B12 in The Vitamins. New York: Academic Press, Inc. 1992.

17. Institute of Medicine. Food and Nutrition Board. Dietary Reference Intakes: Thiamin, Riboflavin, Niacin, Vitamin B6, Folate, Vitamin B12, Pantothenic Acid, Biotin, and Choline. Washington, DC: National Academy Press. 1998.

18. Mackey A, Davis S, Gregory J. Vitamin B6. In: Shils M, Shike M, Ross A, Caballero B, Cousins R, eds. Modern Nutrition in Health and Disease. 10th ed. Baltimore, MD: Lippincott Williams & Wilkins. 2005.

19. Kamen B. Folate and antifolate pharmacology. Semin Oncol. 1997;24:S18-30-S18-39.

20. Bottiglieri T. Folate, vitamin B12, and neuropsychiatric disorders. Nutr Rev. 1996;54:382-90.

21. McCormick D. Vitamin B6. In: Bowman B, Russell R, eds. Present Knowledge in Nutrition. 9th ed. Washington, DC: International Life Sciences Institute. 2006.

22. Jennings E. Folic acid as a cancer preventing agent. Med Hypothesis. 1995;45:297-303.

23. Freudenheim JL, Grahm S, Marshall JR, Haughey BP, Cholewinski S, Wilkinson G. Folate intake and carcinogenesis of the colon and rectum. Int J Epidemiol. 1991;20:368-74.

24. Giovannucci E, Stampfer MJ, Colditz GA, Hunter DJ, Fuchs C, Rosner BA, et al. Multivitamin use, folate, and colon cancer in women in the Nurses' Health Study. Ann Intern Med. 1998;129:517-24.

25. Jacob RA, Sotoudeh G. Vitamin C function and status in chronic disease. Nutr Clin Care. 2002;5:66-74.

26. Frei B, England L, Ames BN. Ascorbate is an outstanding antioxidant in human blood plasma. Proc Natl Acad Sci U S A. 1989;86:6377-81.

27. Carr AC, Frei B. Toward a new recommended dietary allowance for vitamin C based on antioxidant and health effects in humans. Am J Clin Nutr. 1999;69:1086-107.

28. Li Y, Schellhorn HE. New developments and novel therapeutic perspectives for vitamin C. J Nutr. 2007;137:2171-84.

29. Johnston CS, Martin LJ, Cai X. Antihistamine effect of supplemental ascorbic acid and neutrophil chemotaxis. Am Coll Nutr. 1992;11(2):172–6.

30. Clemetson. Histamine and ascorbic acid in human blood. J Nutr. 1980;4(4):662–8.

31. Johnston CS, Solomon RE, Corte C. Vitamin C depletion is associated with alterations in blood histamine and plasma free carnitine in adults. J Am Coll Nutr. 1996;15(6):586–91.

32. Wang AH, Still C. Old world meets modern: a case report of scurvy. Nutr Clin Pract. 2007;22:445-8.

33. Institute of Medicine. Food and Nutrition Board. Dietary Reference Intakes for Vitamin C, Vitamin E, Selenium, and Carotenoids. Washington, DC: National Academy Press. 2000.

34. Francescone MA, Levitt J. Scurvy masquerading as leukocytoclastic vasculitis: a case report and review of the literature. Cutis. 2005;76:261-6.

35. Weinstein M, Babyn P, Zlotkin S. An orange a day keeps the doctor away: scurvy in the year 2000. Pediatrics. 2001;108:E55.

36. Stephen R, Utecht T. Scurvy identified in the emergency department: a case report. J Emerg Med. 2001;21:235-7.

37. Bell EF. History of vitamin E in infant nutrition. Am J Clin Nutr. 1987 Jul;46(1 Suppl):183-6.

38. Traber MG. Vitamin E. In: Shils ME, Shike M, Ross AC, Caballero B, Cousins R, eds. Modern Nutrition in Health and Disease. 10th ed. Baltimore, MD: Lippincott Williams & Wilkins. 2006;396-411.

39. Sokol RJ, Kayden HJ, Bettis DB, Traber MG, Neville H, Ringel S, et al. Isolated vitamin E deficiency in the absence of fat malabsorption—familial and sporadic cases: Characterization and investigation of causes. J Lab Clin Med. 1988 May;111(5):548-59.

40. Laplante P, Vanasse M, Michaud J, Geoffroy G, Brochu P. A progressive neurological syndrome associated with an isolated vitamin E deficiency. Can J Neurol Sci. 1984;11,561-4.

41. Krendel DA, Gilchrest JM, Johnson AO, Bossen EH. Isolated deficiency of vitamin E with progressive neurologic deterioration. Neurology. 1987 Mar;37(3):538-40.

42. Stumpf DA, Sokol R, Bettis D, Neville H, Ringel S, Angelini C, Bell R. Friedreich's disease: V. Variant form with vitamin E deficiency and normal fat absorption. Neurology. 1987;37(1):68-74.

43. Larnaout A, Belal S, Zouari M, Fki M, Ben Hamida C, Goebel, H, et al. Friedreich's ataxia with isolated vitamin E deficiency: a neuropathological study of a Tunisian patient. Acta Neuropathol. 1997 Jun;93(6):633-7.

44. Kohlschütter A, Hubner C, Jansen W, Lindner SG. A treatable familial neuromyopathy with vitamin E deficiency, normal absorption, and evidence of increased consumption of vitamin E. J Inherit Metab Dis. 1988;11 Suppl 2:149-52.

45. Burck U, Goebel HH, Kuhlendahl HD, Meier C, Goebel KM. Neuromyopathy and vitamin E deficiency in man. Neuropediatrics. 1981 Aug;12(3):267-78.

46. Traber MG, Sokol RJ, Ringel SP, Neville HE, Thellman CA, Kayden HJ. Lack of tocopherol in peripheral nerves of vitamin E-deficient patients with peripheral neuropathy. N Engl J Med. 1987 Jul 30;317(5):262-5.

47. Losowsky MS, Leonard PJ. Evidence of vitamin E deficiency in patients with malabsorption or alcoholism and the effects of therapy. Gut. 1967 Dec;8(6):539-43.

48. Farrell P, Bieri J, Fratantoni J, Wood R, Di Sant'Agnese, P. The occurrence and effects of human vitamin E deficiency. A study in patients with cystic fibrosis. J Clin Invest. 1977 Jul;60(1):233-41.

49. Institute of Medicine, Food and Nutrition Board. Dietary Reference Intakes for Calcium and Vitamin D. Washington, DC: National Academy Press. 2010.

50. Cranney C, Horsely T, O'Donnell S, Weiler H, Ooi D, Atkinson S, et al. Effectiveness and safety of vitamin D. Evidence Report/Technology Assessment No. 158 prepared by the University of Ottawa Evidence-based Practice Center under Contract No. 290-02.0021. AHRQ Publication No. 07-E013. Rockville, MD: Agency for Healthcare Research and Quality. 2007.

51. Holick MF. Vitamin D. In: Shils ME, Shike M, Ross AC, Caballero B, Cousins RJ, eds. Modern Nutrition in Health and Disease, 10th ed. Philadelphia: Lippincott Williams & Wilkins. 2006.

52. Norman AW, Henry HH. Vitamin D. In: Bowman BA, Russell RM, eds. Present Knowledge in Nutrition, 9th ed. Washington DC: ILSI Press. 2006.

Image Credits

Index

About the Authors

Sergey A. Dzugan, MD, PhD

Dr. Dzugan is co-founder and Chief Scientific Officer of the Dzugan Institute of Restorative Medicine. Dr. Dzugan graduated from the Donetsk State Medical Institute (Ukraine) with a Doctorate of Medicine in 1979. After medical school, he performed his residency in general and cardiovascular surgery and became the Head of Heart Services in 1985. Dr. Dzugan has had specialized training in vascular surgery, combustiology, microsurgery, arrhythmology, heart surgery, genetic testing, pedagogics, and psychology. Additionally, Dr. Dzugan was a distinguished and highly trained educator, physician, and surgeon in the Ukraine.

In 1990, he received his PhD in Medical Science concerning heart rhythm disorder and subsequently became Assistant Professor at the Donetsk State Medical Institute. In May of 1991, he became the first Chief of the Department of Cardiovascular Surgery and senior Heart Surgeon in Donetsk District Regional Hospital, Ukraine. In March of 1993, he became Associate Professor at Donetsk State Medical University.

Dr. Dzugan has performed a wide spectrum of operations for children and adults, including congenital and acquired heart diseases, as well as rhythm disorders. As the Head of Heart Surgery, he had the highest medical skills and qualifications that could be awarded in his birth country. As a practicing physician, Dr. Dzugan always found himself more in favor of holistic and natural medicines rather than synthetic. He always believed that strengthening one's immune system would do more to improve health than treating problems after they occur. Because of this, while performing heart surgeries, Dr. Dzugan became more interested in the preventive aspects of heart disease and began studying hormone treatments.

Dr. Dzugan moved to the United States from Ukraine in 1995 and, in 1996, became a scientific consultant to Dr. Arnold Smith at the North Central Mississippi Regional Center in Greenwood, Mississippi. His role there was to stay current on the latest advances in nutraceutical treatments with a particular focus on such so as to improve immunity and the ability of patients to fight cancer. Dr. Dzugan has worked with the Cancer Center for more than seven years and was a principle consultant in regards to the Anti-Aging strategy and biological therapy of cancer. The Cancer Center was active in clinical research, and Dr. Dzugan's scholarly background as a clinical researcher helped it proceed in a more organized and scientific fashion. In 1998, he became board certified by the American Academy of Anti-Aging Medicine. His employer at the North Central Mississippi Regional Cancer Center has expressly stated that "Dr. Dzugan is extremely valuable to patient care, and his role differentiates the North Central Mississippi Regional Cancer Center from that of any other centers in the states because no other center has a full-time, well-qualified staff person to meet the same function." Dr. Smith believes that "Dr. Dzugan is a brilliant, gifted physician whose talents we believe would make a significant contribution to the nation."

In 2001, Dr. Dzugan suggested a new hypothesis, hypercholesterolemia, and developed a new statin-free method of high cholesterol treatment. At the same time, he also developed a unique multimodal program for migraine management.

In October 2003, he moved to Ft. Lauderdale, Florida, and became the Manager of the Advisory Department at the Life Extension Foundation. Later, he became President of Life Extension Scientific Information, Inc. In August 2006, Dr. Dzugan left the Life Extensions Foundation to create a scientific organization that consults physicians on how to develop the program for their patients in order to optimize physiology.

Dr. Dzugan was accepted (June, 30 2006) to the International Academy of Creative Endeavors (Moscow, Russia) as a Corresponding Member of the Academy for his outstanding contribution to the development of new methods of hypercholesterolemia and migraine treatment. One year later, the Academy awarded Dr. Dzugan with the honorary title of "Academician." In December 2007, Dr. Dzugan was rewarded with an Honoree Medal by this Academy for his personal input into the physical betterment of nations and the strengthening of friendships between them, as well as their acquisition of science and culture,. He performed presentations multiple times at the prestigious International Congress on Anti-Aging Medicine. The topics of his presentations were related to cholesterol disorders, migraines, physiology optimization, stem cell therapy, cancer, and immunorestorative and hormonorestorative therapies.

Dr. Dzugan is the author of 151 medical journal publications, and these publications include surgical, oncological, academic, and anti-aging topics. Also, several articles were published in health-related magazines, such as *Life Extension Magazine* and *The South African Journal of Natural Medicine*. He is the author of the following books: *Migraine Cure, Dzugan Method | Restorative Medicine, The Magic of Cholesterol Numbers,* and *Your Blood Doesn't Lie!* and is also the holder of three heart-surgery-related patents. Dr. Dzugan is a Member of the Editorial Board of the

Neuroendocrinology Letters and a member of the Medical Advisory Board at *Life Extension Magazine*. He is co-founder and President of iPOMS (International Physiology Optimization Medical Society).

Dr. Dzugan's current primary interests are physiologic therapy for elevated cholesterol, migraines, fatigue, fibromyalgia, and behavioral and hormonal disorders.

Konstantine S. Dzugan

Konstantine is a scientific advisor of the Dzugan Institute of Restorative Medicine. Konstantine graduated from Florida Atlantic University in 2010.

He is the author of two medical journal publications, as well as of one book. His primary interests include: the development of programs for the optimization of physiology, botanical wizardry via the creation of chlorophyll-rich biomass, explorations of drowned coasts, collection of semi-precious stones, research on lost cultures, and writing out inadequate extended metaphors.

THE
RESTORATION
OF THE
HUMAN BODY

[IN 7 PARTS]

SECOND EDITION

For more information please visit us on the web:
www.DzLogic.com
or contact us at 866-225-4877.